A Guide to NIH Grant Programs

A Guide to
NIH Grant Programs

Samuel M. Schwartz, Ph.D.

Mischa E. Friedman, Ph.D.

New York   Oxford
OXFORD UNIVERSITY PRESS
1992

MAR 9 4

Oxford University Press

Oxford   New York   Toronto
Delhi   Bombay   Calcutta   Madras   Karachi
Kuala Lumpur   Singapore   Hong Kong   Tokyo
Nairobi   Dar es Salaam   Cape Town
Melbourne   Auckland

and associated companies in
Berlin   Ibadan

Published by Oxford University Press, Inc.,
200 Madison Avenue, New York, New York 10016

Oxford is a registered trademark of Oxford University Press

Library of Congress Cataloging-in-Publication Data
Schwartz, Samuel M.
A guide to NIH grant programs / Samuel M. Schwartz, Mischa E. Friedman.
p. cm.   Includes bibliographical references.
ISBN 0-19-506934-X
1. National Institutes of Health (U.S.)—Research grants.
2. Federal aid to medical research—United States.
I. Friedman, Mischa E.   II. Title.
[DNLM: 1. National Institutes of Health (U.S.)
2. Research Support—organization & administration—United States—handbooks.
W 39 S399g]   RA11.D6S38   1992
610'.79'73—dc20   DNLM/DLC   for Library of Congress   92-6084

9 8 7 6 5 4 3 2 1

Printed in the United States of America
on acid-free paper

Preface

There is a vast amount of material available describing the extramural grants review and award process at the National Institutes of Health (NIH). We have undertaken to write this book to organize and highlight the most significant information about the NIH grants programs. Our purpose is to assist members of the biomedical and behavioral research communities in understanding the inner workings of the system and to facilitate their pursuit of research support.

We would like to thank the NIH, especially the Division of Research Grants (DRG), for furnishing information, tables, and figures from their many publications. We are grateful for the input of our many colleagues and former associates at NIH. We especially want to thank Drs. Samuel Joseloff and Miriam Kelty of the NIH and Dr. Halvor Aaslestad of Yale University for reviewing our manuscript and for their many helpful comments. Thanks also are due to Edith Barry, Susan Hannan, and Ginger Wineinger, our editors at Oxford University Press, for their guidance and to our former editor, Dr. Alasdair J. Ritchie, whose enthusiasm for the project is appreciated. Our gratitude also is extended to Dr. Daniel Lufkin for his excellent technical advice and assistance. Finally, the input from our wives, Myra Helman Schwartz and Greta Zimmer Friedman, was valuable, as was their patience, support, and encouragement, which made the project a more pleasant experience.

Chevy Chase, Md.   S.M.S.
Frederick, Md.   M.E.F.
February 1992

Authors' Note

The National Institutes of Health (NIH) was in no way connected with this project. The sole responsibility for its content, its factual material, and interpretation of policies and procedures resides with the authors. We have attempted to include the most current information and data. However, it should be recognized that the programs of NIH are dynamic. New policies, procedures, and mechanisms of support are constantly being developed and may not be described in this book because of publication schedules. For example, the research components of the three Alcohol, Drug Abuse, and Mental Health Administration (ADAMHA) institutes may become part of NIH. Information about these institutes has not been included but can be obtained by contacting the following offices at 5600 Fishers Lane, Rockville, MD 20857:

> National Institute on Alcohol Abuse and Alcoholism
> Office of Scientific Affairs
> Room 16C-20, Parklawn Building
> (301) 443-4375

> National Institute on Drug Abuse
> Office of Extramural Program Review
> Room 10-42, Parklawn Building
> (301) 443-2755

> National Institute of Mental Health
> Division of Extramural Activities
> Room 9-105, Parklawn Building
> (301) 443-3367

We do acknowledge the extensive use, in whole or in part, of the content of NIH documents, which are available to the public. In some cases, sections of such documents have been used unchanged to ensure the accuracy of the information being transmitted. However, reference to the source document is made in appropriate places in the book.

S.M.S.
M.E.F.

Contents

Abbreviations

ADAMHA	Alcohol, Drug Abuse, and Mental Health Administration
AHR	Ad hoc review
AIDS	Acquired Immunodeficiency Syndrome
ARA	Awaiting receipt of application
AREA	Academic Research Enhancement Award
BRSG	Biomedical Research Support Grant
CC	Clinical center
CIA	Clinical Investigator Award
DCRT	Division of Computer Research and Technology
DDER	Deputy Director for Extramural Research
DHHS	Department of Health and Human Services
DRG	Division of Research Grants
FIC	Fogarty International Center
FIRST	First Independent Research Support and Transition Award
FOIA	Freedom of Information Act
FY	Fiscal year
HPP	High program priority
IACUC	Institutional Animal Care and Use Committee
ICD	Institutes, Centers, and Divisions
IRB	Institutional Review Board
ISB/DRG	Information Systems Branch, Division of Research Grants
IRG	Initial Review Group
LPP	Low program priority
MARC	Minority Access to Research Careers
MBRS	Minority Biomedical Research Support
MERIT	Method to Extend Research in Time
MSTP	Medical Sciences Training Program
NCHGR	National Center for Human Genome Research
NCI	National Cancer Institute
NCNR	National Center for Nursing Research
NCRR	National Center for Research Resources
NEI	National Eye Institute
NHLBI	National Heart, Lung, and Blood Institute
NIA	National Institute on Aging
NIAID	National Institute of Allergy and Infectious Diseases

NIAMS	National Institute of Arthritis and Musculoskeletal and Skin Diseases
NICHD	National Institute of Child Health and Human Development
NIDCD	National Institute on Deafness and Other Communication Disorders
NIDDK	National Institute of Diabetes and Digestive and Kidney Diseases
NIDR	National Institute of Dental Research
NIEHS	National Institute of Environmental Health Sciences
NIGMS	National Institute of General Medical Sciences
NIH	National Institutes of Health
NINDS	National Institute of Neurological Disorders and Stroke
NLM	National Library of Medicine
NRSA	National Research Service Award
OASH	Office of the Assistant Secretary for Health
OD/NIH	Office of the Director, National Institutes of Health
OIG	Outstanding Investigator Grant
OMB	Office of Management and Budget
OPRR	Office for Protection from Research Risks
PA	Privacy Act
PA	Program Announcement
PHS	Public Health Service
PSA	Physician Scientist Award
PI	Principal Investigator
PSV	Project site visit
RCDA	Research Career Development Award
RCMI	Research Centers in Minority Institutions
RFA	Request for Applications
RFP	Request for Proposals
RPG	Research Project Grant
RRB/DRG	Referral and Review Branch, Division of Research Grants
SBIR	Small Business Innovation Research
SCOR	Specialized Centers of Research
SEP	Special Emphasis Panel
SRA	Scientific Review Administrator (formerly Executive Secretary)
SRG	Scientific Review Group
SS	Study Section
SSS	Special Study Section
USPHS	United States Public Health Service

A Guide to NIH Grant Programs

1

Introduction

The National Institutes of Health (NIH) is the premier biomedical research organization in the world. It serves as the U.S. government's lead agency in the war on human disease. It carries out its mission of providing leadership and research direction to biomedical research programs through its clinics, in-house laboratory research, and extramural programs. In doing so, NIH is the largest supporter of biomedical research in the country. Of its total budget of over $8 billion in fiscal year (FY) 1991, over 80 percent was allocated for the support of extramural grants and contracts. These are awarded to thousands of institutions and scientists around the world, but mostly in the United States.

Each year approximately 40,000 biomedical and behavioral researchers apply to the United States Public Health Service (USPHS) for support of their research or research training, with the vast majority of applications submitted to the NIH.

The NIH is located in Bethesda, Maryland, and consists of 21 institutes, centers, and divisions (ICDs). One institute, the National Institute on Aging, has its intramural laboratories in Baltimore and another, the National Institute of Environmental Health Sciences, resides in the Research Triangle Park, North Carolina. Eighteen ICDs support research and research training through grants and contracts with funds awarded and administered by their extramural programs.

Of the many who apply for support, at least 60 percent are first-time applicants seeking to establish careers in research. Many of these investigators, and indeed even some experienced researchers, know little of the structure and organization of NIH. They may be unaware of the complexities of the extramural programs, of the peer review system used to process and evaluate their grant applications, and of how decisions are made.

As managers in the peer review system, we were often asked: "What is the most useful advice you could offer members of the biomedical and behavioral research communities?" We invariably answered that it is essential for an investigator to know and understand—free of rumors, innuendo, and gossip—the NIH peer review system; what it is, how it operates, who peoples it, and what its limitations are. In addition, it is essential to know and understand how the programs are managed, the available types of awards, the research and research training support programs, and how best to prepare grant applications.

This book is meant to supplement, not replace, the instructions that accompany the various federal application forms. Its purpose is to bring to researchers and administrators, especially the beginning investigator, the most useful, straightforward information to aid them in their quest for support. Also, we hope that in supplying this information, we can help the applicants avoid delays in the processing of applications. In organizing this book, our intent is to:

- Provide information about the NIH, its organizational structure, and the missions and budgets of its component parts
- Define specifically the large variety of extramural award mechanisms and programs available to support research, research training, and related activities
- Provide guidance in the preparation of applications for competitive consideration by the NIH
- Indicate whom to talk with at NIH and at the investigator's institution
- Describe the scientific evaluation procedures leading to award decisions, highlighting the various decision points in the process. The main focus is on the well-known NIH peer review system.
- Provide information on the management of awards by the NIH program staff
- Identify a variety of useful sources of information about the extramural programs
- Include insights into the granting process from the perspective of the authors' past experiences

As the research community has come to realize, the availability of NIH funding is unpredictable and subject to many variables. Funding priorities may shift, with AIDS research and the Human Genome Research Project currently receiving much attention. In addition, the number of grant awards the NIH can make has fluctuated, with a serious decline in recent fiscal years. Some of this has been due to the increase in the number of applications submitted, the increase in the cost of doing research, the increase in the number of mechanisms of support, as well as an increase in funds earmarked for special initiatives, and an increased use of the Request for Applications (RFAs).

The one unshakable constant that remains is the formidable competitiveness of the process. While a meritorious idea carried out as good science is still the essential ingredient in acquiring support, it may not be sufficient if the application is inadequately prepared or if the decision-making process is not understood. Thus, by providing an abundance of practical and useful information about the NIH extramural programs and processes, we hope this book will assist investigators in gaining a more favorable edge in obtaining support for their research programs.

2

NIH Mission and Organization

As of the end of February, 1992 the National Institutes of Health's "Framework for Discussion of Strategies for NIH" defined the agency's mission, goals, and objectives in the following way:*

NIH MISSION STATEMENT

Science in pursuit of knowledge to extend healthy life and reduce the burdens of illness and disability.

NIH GOALS

1. To foster innovative research strategies designed to advance significantly the nation's capacity to improve health.
2. To provide the scientific base that will strengthen the nation's capability to deliver more effective disease prevention and health care in order to enhance the quality of its citizens lives.
3. To expand the knowledge base in biomedical and behavioral research in order to enhance the nation's economic competitiveness and ensure a continued high return on the public investment in research.
4. To exemplify and promote public accountability, scientific integrity, and social responsibility.

NIH OBJECTIVES

1. Critical science and technology: Assure that critical science and technology in basic biology impacting on human health and the national economy are advanced as priorities across NIH.
2. Research capacity: Strengthen the capacity of the national biomedical and behavioral research enterprise to respond to current and emerging public health needs.

*From *Chemical and Engineering News,* March 9, 1992.

3. Intellectual capital: Provide for the renewal and growth of the intellectual capital base essential to the biomedical research enterprise. Ensuring fairness and equality of opportunity at NIH is central to efforts to enhance the human resource base of biomedical research.
4. Stewardship of public resources: Secure the maximal return on the public investment in the enterprise.
5. Public trust: Continually earn the public's respect, trust, and confidence as we carry out our mission.

The NIH campus in Bethesda is located on a 306-acre site. More than fifty buildings house the intramural research laboratories, the research hospital known as the Warren Grant Magnuson Clinical Center, the Office of the Director and the headquarters' staff, and the offices and staff of most of the institute directors. While there are a number of off-campus facilities in the Washington metropolitan area and elsewhere, at least one satellite office building is deserving of special attention. The Westwood Building, 5333 Westbard Avenue, Bethesda, is the home of the Division of Research Grants (DRG) and the extramural staff of several of the institutes. The main campus is easily accessible by subway from the Washington National Airport or Union Station. From the campus, shuttle buses run on regular schedules to the Westwood and other NIH office buildings in the Bethesda area.

The NIH is part of the Department of Health and Human Services (DHHS). It is one of the health agencies within the Department's United States Public Health Service (USPHS). The main components of the NIH are institutes, centers, and divisions (ICDs). Table 2.1 is a simplified depiction of the organization and its place in the DHHS hierarchy.

The emphasis in Table 2.1 is on the NIH units that fund grant and contract proposals. All of the listed components do, with the exception of the DRG. It is included because of its key role in the NIH extramural programs.

The DRG has a number of important responsibilities related to the NIH grants program. It has no involvement with the contract programs except for data management and analysis. Its most significant functions are to:

- Serve as the central receipt, assignment, and referral point for all grant applications submitted to the NIH. It also performs the same service for other Public Health Service agencies, e.g., ADAMHA
- Provide scientific review of most, but not all, NIH grant applications
- Collect and analyze data on the NIH extramural programs for internal management purposes and for dissemination to the scientific community and the public
- Offer advice and staff support to the institutes and the Office of the Director, NIH, in formulating grant policies and procedures

Particular emphasis is given to the first two of these functions in the chapters to follow.

TABLE 2.1. NIH Organization

Office of the Secretary, DHHS

Assistant Secretary for Health

Public Health Service (PHS)

(Surgeon General)

Agency for Health Care Policy and Research

Agency for Toxic Substances and Disease Registry

Alcohol, Drug Abuse, and Mental Health Administration

Centers for Disease Control

Food and Drug Administration

Indian Health Service

Health Resources and Services Administration

National Institutes of Health

Institutes
National Institute on Aging (NIA)

National Institute of Allergy and Infectious Diseases (NIAID)

National Institute of Arthritis and Musculoskeletal and Skin Diseases (NIAMS)

National Cancer Institute (NCI)

National Institute of Child Health and Human Development (NICHD)

National Institute on Deafness and Other Communication Disorders (NIDCD)

National Institute of Dental Research (NIDR)

National Institute of Diabetes and Digestive and Kidney Diseases (NIDDK)

National Institute of Environmental Health Sciences (NIEHS)

National Eye Institute (NEI)

National Institute of General Medical Sciences (NIGMS)

National Heart, Lung, and Blood Institute (NHLBI)

National Institute of Neurological Disorders and Stroke (NINDS)

National Library of Medicine (NLM)

Centers
Fogarty International Center (FIC)

National Center for Human Genome Research (NCHGR)

National Center for Nursing Research (NCNR)

National Center for Research Resources (NCRR)

Divisions
Division of Research Grants (DRG)

In addition to the organization of NIH as a whole, it is instructive to describe the structure of an individual institute. Although there are many internal variations, a common pattern exists. Every institute has an advisory council or board, analogous to a board of directors, to provide advice on grant recommendations and fiscal and policy issues relevant to the institute's affairs. Most institutes have both intramural and extramural programs. The exceptions are the National Institute of General Medical Sciences (NIGMS), and the Fogarty International Center (FIC), which support no intramural activities. The other institutes carry on both laboratory and clinical research intramurally. A board of scientific counselors, composed of non-federal scientists, peer reviews an institute's intramural research efforts and advises on the quality of the programs and staff on a regular basis.

An institute's extramural program, in a sense, is modeled after the NIH structure. There are several disease-oriented program areas, each a discrete unit responsible for the scientific management of grant and contract programs. In addition, there is a service division, such as a division of extramural affairs, to perform functions required by all program areas. These would include peer review of special grant and contract proposals, contract and grant management activities, development and coordination of extramural policies and procedures, and a number of important support services such as managing committee and council affairs, maintaining mail and file rooms, and the institute's extramural data system. The accompanying chart describes the typical institute organization.

Office of the Institute Director: National Advisory Council/Board

Intramural Programs: Board of Scientific Counselors
Laboratory studies

Clinical studies

Extramural Programs
Program divisions

Division or Office of Extramural Affairs

PROGRAM INTERESTS OF THE INDIVIDUAL NIH INSTITUTES

In addition to the general statement of the mission of the NIH, a more detailed picture of the scientific and disease interests of each of the NIH institutes that award grants and contracts should prove useful. Although the name of an institute is obviously suggestive of its mission, potential grant applicants may be surprised to learn of the breadth of interests and the willingness to support a broad spectrum of basic science research. The sections that follow for each institute are by no means complete and in some cases may be dated because of the rapidly changing nature of science and research priorities.

A brief abstract and key word descriptors are used to indicate the special program interests of the various NIH funding components. The institute program staff should be contacted for additional information.

NATIONAL INSTITUTE ON AGING (NIA)

The NIA supports biomedical, social, and behavioral research and training related to the aging process, diseases, and other special problems of the aged. Interests are in fundamental studies of biological processes, as well as in clinical processes such as Alzheimer's disease, osteoporosis, osteoarthritis, falls, and urinary incontinence. Research programs also are concerned with the psychological, cultural, and economic factors that affect both the aging process and the roles of older people in society. Some relevant key word descriptors are listed in the accompanying chart.

Cell biology	Retirement
Molecular biology	Clinical problems of the elderly
Genetics of aging	Behavioral geriatrics
Musculoskeletal systems	Pharmacology and aging
Animal models	Biopsychological aging
Neurobiology of aging	Cognitive, sensory, psychomotor processes of aging
Dementias of aging	
Sensory processes	Social and psychological factors in aging
Sleep disorders of the aged	
Exercise and aging	The elderly in social institutions
Nutrition, metabolism, and GI tract function	Societal aspects of aging
Immunology and aging	Methodological studies
Endocrinology	General longitudinal studies
Cardiovascular, pulmonary, and hematologic function in aging	Research related to health services for the elderly

NATIONAL INSTITUTE OF ALLERGY AND INFECTIOUS DISEASES (NIAID)

The programs emphasize fundamental and clinical investigations of the immune system; and all forms of prevention, diagnosis, therapy, and epidemiology of viral, bacterial, fungal, and parasitic diseases.

- Asthma and other allergic diseases
- Structure and function of the immune system
- Immunogenetics and transplantation biology
- Clinical immunology and immunopathology
- Infectious diseases and the host response
- Bacterial and fungal diseases

- Viral diseases
- Parasitic diseases
- Molecular microbiology
- Treatment of AIDS, including preclinical drug development
- Prevention of AIDS
- Epidemiology of AIDS
- Pathogenesis of AIDS

NATIONAL INSTITUTE OF ARTHRITIS, MUSCULOSKELETAL, AND SKIN DISEASES (NIAMS)

The NIAMS supports research on connective tissue, bone, muscle, skin, and cartilage and including arthritis, rheumatic diseases, skin diseases, and orthopedics. The emphasis is on clinical and basic studies on structure and function, etiology, epidemiology, pathogenesis, diagnosis, treatment, prevention, and control of specific diseases and disorders:

- Structure, function, physiology, and development of connective tissue, joints, muscle, bone, and skin
- Rheumatic and connective tissue diseases and disorders
- Skin diseases and disorders
- Bone diseases and disorders
- Muscle and its diseases and disorders
- Epidemiological and behavioral research related to connective tissue, joints, muscle, bone, and skin

NATIONAL CANCER INSTITUTE (NCI)

The NCI sponsors laboratory and clinical investigations relating to the cause, prevention, diagnosis, and treatment of cancer. It also funds research in cancer control, rehabilitation, education, and training. These areas are listed below:

- Diagnosis
- Immunology
- Biological carcinogenesis
- Chemical/physical carcinogenesis
- Biometry
- Epidemiology
- Special emphasis areas:
    - Biochemical epidemiology
    - Diet—nutrition epidemiology
    - AIDS epidemiology

- Biochemistry and pharmacology
- Clinical treatment
- Radiation therapy
- Diagnostic imaging
- Low-level radiation effects
- Biological response modifiers
- Nutrition
- Surgical oncology
- Prevention
- Community oncology
- Health promotion sciences
- Evaluation and cancer control

NATIONAL INSTITUTE ON DEAFNESS AND OTHER COMMUNICATION DISORDERS (NIDCD)

Areas of concern are hearing and deafness, balance and the vestibular system, voice, taste, smell, language, speech, and touch:

- Speech, language, and cognitive disorders
- Speech and language processes
- Hearing and vestibular function
- Taste, smell, and chemical sense
- Sensory mechanisms
- Prostheses

NATIONAL INSTITUTE OF DENTAL RESEARCH (NIDR)

The mission of the NIDR is to fund research related to the etiology, pathogenesis, diagnosis, treatment, and prevention of dental and orofacial diseases and conditions:

- Normal teeth
- Dental caries and erosion of tooth crowns and roots
- Acquired craniofacial defects
- Bone formation and remodeling related to craniofacial structures
- Dental caries prevention
- Restorative materials
- Periodontal diseases
- Oral cancer
- Salivary glands and their secretions
- Oral soft tissues
- Artificial dental implants; transplantation and replantation of natural teeth

- Developmental biology of the craniofacial complex
- Craniofacial anomalies
- Malocclusion and craniofacial growth
- Geriatric dentistry
- Psychological aspects of oral diseases
- Behavioral aspects of oral health care
- Neurobiological bases of orofacial and dental pain
- Diagnosis and treatment of orofacial and dental pain
- Diagnosis, treatment, and neurobiological bases of orofacial motor and sensory function and dysfunction, including taste and smell

NATIONAL INSTITUTE OF DIABETES AND DIGESTIVE AND KIDNEY DISEASES (NIDDK)

The NIDDK supports research on diabetes, endocrinology, metabolism, and metabolic diseases; nutrition, eating disorders, obesity, and the organ systems and components associated with the gastrointestinal tract; and renal diseases, urology, and hematology:

- Nature, function, and action of hormones, brain–gut peptides, and hormonelike agents
- Endocrine systems and their disorders
- Insulin and other agents for control of blood glucose
- Fundamental and clinical nutrition in diabetes mellitus
- Diseases and disorders of the exocrine pancreas, biliary tract and liver, and experimental models
- Fundamental and clinical nutrition, malnutrition, patho-physiology, nutrient metabolism
- Clinical and fundamental studies of obesity, eating disorders, and energy regulation
- Causative and exacerbating factors of diabetes mellitus
- Normal/abnormal metabolic processes
- Metabolic diseases and disorders
- Cystic fibrosis
- Structure and function of the organ systems of the GI tract
- Diseases and disorders of GI organ systems and experimental models
- Intestinal immunology and inflammatory diseases
- Structure/ function of the exocrine, pancreas, biliary tract, and liver
- Renal physiology, pathophysiology, and cell biology
- Renal failure, end-stage renal disease, and maintenance therapies for renal disease

- Urological diseases and disorders
- Hematopoiesis and factors affecting its control and regulation
- Hematologic disorders and therapeutic modalities
- Tissue and organ transplantation

NATIONAL INSTITUTE OF ENVIRONMENTAL HEALTH SCIENCES (NIEHS)

The NIEHS supports research and training on the biological effects of environmental chemicals and physical factors, as listed below. These terms are interpreted broadly to include chemicals and agents to which humans are exposed in work, home, and recreational/leisure environments via air, water, food, and skin contact. They include such materials as cleansing chemicals and smoke components; socioenvironmental agents such as food additives, consumer chemicals, and air and water pollutants; and ambient agents such as sunlight and natural food contaminants. Thus, there is interest in the study of all agents in the environment (chemical, physical, and biological) that produce an obvious and suspected biological effect which may impinge upon human health. Interest extends from the molecular and cellular levels to the organ and organismic levels, and to human populations. The endpoints may be represented by a diversity of specific disease entities, such as neurologic disorders, chronic fibrocystic disease, cancer, and so forth, through the less obvious subtle changes that occur at the cellular and molecular levels. Alternatives to the traditional methods for assessing or predicting the toxicity of environmental agents, such as microbial and nonmammalian species, are of special interest.

- Biological effects of environmental agents and their mechanism of action
- Method and toxicological test development
- Human health effects, laboratory and epidemiological investigations
- Aquatic species as models for human environmental health processes/ toxicological effects
- Alternatives in toxicity testing.

NATIONAL EYE INSTITUTE (NEI)

The NEI supports research on the normal function, structure, and development of the eye, vision, and the visual system; causes of disorders of the eye, vision, and the visual system; the prevention, diagnosis, and treatment of these disorders, and to enhance the rehabilitation, training, and quality of life of blind and partially sighted persons:

- Blindness and low vision
- Cornea and external eye
- Visual nervous system
- Eye muscles and movement
- Lens and cataract
- Aqueous humor, vitreous humor, and uvea
- Glaucoma
- Retina and choroid
- Vision and visual function
- Specific eye complications of systemic disorders

NATIONAL INSTITUTE OF GENERAL MEDICAL SCIENCES (NIGMS)

The principal goal of the NIGMS is to support basic and clinical research that complements the missions of the disease-oriented institutes, as follows:

- Biophysics of proteins and nucleic acids
- Chromosome mapping, DNA sequencing
- DNA replication, mutagenesis
- Chromosomal structure and mechanics
- Extrachromosomal inheritance
- Gene expression, RNA, and protein synthesis
- Bioenergetics
- Receptors
- Drug interactions
- Toxic effects of therapeutic drugs
- Drug disposition
- Drug metabolism
- Clinical pharmacology
- Anesthesiology research
- Population genetics and complex genetic systems
- Developmental genetics
- Medical genetics
- Cell structure and function
- Cell division and the cycle
- Regulation of development, cell differentiation, and growth
- Membrane structure and function
- Cellular and molecular biology of model cell systems
- Molecular basis of enzyme catalysis and regulation
- Medicinal chemistry

- Physiological and biochemical responses to trauma, including burn injury
- Basic biological mechanisms of behavior and adaptation
- Biomedical engineering
- Instrument development

NATIONAL INSTITUTE OF CHILD HEALTH AND HUMAN DEVELOPMENT (NICHD)

The NICHD's programs include basic and clinical research relating to maternal and child health and human development, reproduction, population dynamics, developmental biology, clinical nutrition, perinatal and infant morbidity and mortality, and mental retardation and developmental disabilities. Generally, these are biological and behavioral studies of normal and abnormal growth, development, and maturation from gametogenesis through maturity.

- Reproductive biology
- Reproductive chemistry and endocrinology
- Reproductive genetics and immunology
- Reproductive medicine
- Fertility, infertility, family planning, and fertility regulation
- Demographic, social, and behavioral population sciences
- Sudden infant death syndrome
- Nutrition: biomedical and behavioral
- Pediatric and developmental neuro- and endocrinology
- Biological bases of behavioral development
- Learning, cognition, and communicative abilities
- Population research methodology
- Population structure, distribution, and migration
- Pregnancy and labor
- Fetal pathophysiology/development
- Perinatology
- Developmental and clinical genetics
- Embryogenesis, developmental biology, and teratology
- Developmental immunology
- Social and affective development
- Family studies
- Behavioral pediatrics
- Childhood injury
- Mental retardation and developmental disabilities
- AIDS: reproductive, pediatric, and behavioral aspects
- Rehabilitation

NATIONAL HEART, LUNG, AND BLOOD INSTITUTE (NHLBI)

The NHLBI is committed to support research and training related to the normal structure and function, and disease or dysfunction, of the cardiovascular, respiratory, and blood systems. Broad interests can be summarized as follows:

- Basic, applied, and clinical research
- Molecular and cellular biology
- Control mechanisms
- Genetics
- Normal functions
- Etiology and pathogenesis
- Clinical trials
- Demonstration and education

More specific program interests include:

- Arteriosclerosis
- Coronary heart disease
- Cardiac diseases, cardiomyopathies, myocarditis
- Congenital heart diseases
- Rheumatic heart disease
- Sudden death
- Peripheral vascular disease
- Cerebrovascular disease
- Structure and function of the respiratory system
- Pediatric pulmonary diseases
- Occupational and immunological pulmonary disease
- Chronic diseases of the airways
- Pulmonary vascular diseases
- Respiratory failure
- Coagulation, fibrinolysis, and thrombosis
- Development, structure, and function, of the cardiovascular system
- Behavioral aspects of heart, lung, and blood diseases
- Hypertension and kidney disease
- Cardiovascular aspects of diabetes mellitus
- Devices, technology, protheses and biomaterials, therapeutic and diagnostic instrumentation
- Epidemiological research related to heart, lung, and blood diseases
- Nutrition and diet as related to heart, lung, and blood diseases
- Hemorrhagic disorders
- Platelets and megakaryocytes

- Red blood cell membranes
- Sickle cell disease, thalassemia (Cooley's anemia), and other hereditary hemoglobinopathies
- Hematopoiesis, aplastic anemia
- Blood components, derivatives, and substitutes
- Transfusion medicine
- Tissue and organ transplantation and storage
- Prevention and control
- Childhood precursors of heart and lung disease in adults
- Smoking, health effects

NATIONAL LIBRARY OF MEDICINE (NLM)

The NLM supports research in the organization, representation, utilization, and dissemination of health information, and in the development of health information resources, services, and systems. Such research includes linguistics, bibliographies, databases, knowledge bases, information transfer, and the use of symbolically expressed knowledge for problem-solving and decision-making strategies.

- Medical informatics (computers in medicine)
- Computer-based representation and analysis of molecular biology data
- Medical (health sciences) libraries
- Medical (health) knowledge utilization
- Integrated medical information management
- Medical knowledge organization
- Preparation and/or publication of nonprofit scholarly or scientific literary projects

NATIONAL CENTER FOR NURSING RESEARCH (NCNR)

The NCNR supports nursing research and research training related to patient care, the promotion of health, the prevention of disease, and the mitigation of acute and chronic illnesses and disabilities:

- Health promotion and disease prevention
- Acute and chronic illness
- Nursing systems
- Ethics of patient care
- Patient care of HIV-infected individuals, AIDS patients, and their families

NATIONAL INSTITUTE OF NEUROLOGICAL DISORDERS AND STROKE (NINDS)

The NINDS supports research on the nervous system, with major emphasis on studies of the cerebrovascular system the neuromuscular system, and neuropsychology. Specific areas include epidemiology, etiology, and pathogenesis; investigations of diagnosis, treatment, prevention, and control, including rehabilitation; and clinical trials.

- Stroke and other cerebrovascular diseases and disorders
- Convulsive and related episodic states, including sleep
- Demyelinating and immunologically mediated disorders of the nervous system
- Genetic disorders of the nervous system
- Neuroendocrine studies
- Neural aspects of learning, perception, and memory
- Neural prostheses
- Degenerative disorders of the nervous system
- Muscular, neuromuscular, and peripheral nerve disorders
- AIDS and other retrovirus-associated neurological disorders of humans and animals
- Infectious disorders of the nervous system
- Trauma and injury to the nervous system (central and peripheral)
- Nervous system regeneration
- Primary tumors of the nervous system
- Nutritional deficiencies that affect the nervous system
- Neurotoxicology
- Developmental neurobiology and neurological disorders of early life
- Movement disorders
- Dementias and neurological disorders of adult life
- Imaging and monitoring of the nervous system
- Autonomic nervous system, function and disorders

NATIONAL CENTER FOR RESEARCH RESOURCES (NCRR)

The NCRR supports institutional, regional, and national research resources and resource-related research projects:

- Animal research
- Biomedical research technology
- General clinical research

- Research facilities improvement
- Shared instrumentation

NATIONAL CENTER FOR HUMAN GENOME RESEARCH (NCHGR)

The NCHGR mission is to characterize the structure of the human genome. The primary objective is the development of genetic and physical maps in human and model organisms, the acquisition of the entire DNA sequence of those genomes, and the development of new technology to achieve these goals. Because of the extensive amount of information available about the genetics and molecular biology of *Escherichia coli*, *Saccharomyces cerevisiae*, *Drosophila melanogaster*, *Caenorhabditis elegans*, and *Mus musculus*, there is particular interest in these models. If others are to be used, a clear rationale and relationship to the genome program is expected.

- Genetic and physical mapping
- DNA sequencing
- Technology development
- Data and materials management
- Ethical, legal, and social issues

FOGARTY INTERNATIONAL CENTER (FIC)

The FIC is responsible for furthering international cooperation and collaboration by supporting biomedical and behavioral research, development of research manpower, and the prevention of disease and improvement of health worldwide:

- Fellowships/training grants that promote collaboration and cooperation internationally
- Research and conferences that promote cooperation, collaboration, and the transfer of research results internationally

3

Budget and Legislation

The legislative process which mainly affects NIH involves appropriations (budgeting funds) and authorizations (permission to carry out individual programs). Not only are these done by separate acts of Congress, but the bills are considered and recommended by separate committees of Congress.

The individual components of NIH independently develop their budget requests according to previous commitments, current activities, future program plans and priorities, and resource requirements. The requests are reviewed and approved by the Office of the Director, NIH (OD/NIH), and the total NIH budget is then sent forward to the USPHS, the Office of the Assistant Secretary for Health (OASH) of the DHHS, and the Office of Management and Budget (OMB). After these offices approve the request, usually with modifications, the President submits the budget to the Congress. While all the components of NIH go through this route, the current law permits the NCI to submit its request as a bypass budget directly to the President. However, in practice, the NCI joins with the other ICDs in following the traditional budget process.

The NIH differs from most other federal agencies in that annually each institute presents and defends its own budget before the following committees of the Congress: (1) the Labor, Health and Human Services, Education, and Related Agencies Subcommittee of the House Committee on Appropriations and (2) the Labor, Health and Human Services, Education, and Related Agencies Subcommittee of the Senate Committee on Appropriations. Members from the 102nd Congress (1991–93) are listed in Tables 3.1 and 3.2. Published proceedings from these hearings are informative and can be obtained from the Government Printing Office (for a fee), the Committee Office (must be picked up in person), or from one's congressional representative (may or may not be mailed).

Thus, monies are not appropriated to the NIH as a whole. Instead, funds are appropriated by specific budgetary legislation directly to the institutes and distributed within them to support their many programs and activities. Of course, Congress frequently mandates sums of money to be spent on specific programs, e.g., AIDS or specific genetic diseases, and the particular ICD must use those funds in the fiscal year(s) designated. It is important to remember, however, that appropri-

TABLE 3.1. Labor, Health and Human Services,
Education and Related Agencies Subcommittee
of the House Committee on Appropriations

Majority Members	Minority Members
William Natcher, KY (Chairman)	Carl Pursell, MI (Ranking)
Neal Smith, IA	John Porter, IL
David Obey, WI	C. W. Bill Young, FL
Edward Roybal, CA	Vin Weber, MN
Louis Stokes, OH	
Joseph Early, MA	
Steny Hoyer, MD	
Robert Mrazek, NY	

ated funds cannot be spent unless Congress also authorizes the programs of NIH in separate legislation and the OMB allocates the money.

The aggregate NIH budget consists of line items of the various mechanisms of extramural support, intramural research, and internal support activities. These are detailed in Table 3.3, which shows that of the FY 1991 allowance of $8.3 billion, approximately 80 percent was designated for extramural grant and contract programs. However, it is important to understand that all of this money does not go for the award of new grants. Of the $6.6 billion that was earmarked for the extramural programs, $4.9 billion or 74.1 percent was set aside for noncompeting projects, which represented NIH's commitment base. This sum was for the second, third, fourth, or fifth years of already awarded grants and contracts.

While the aggregate NIH budget deals with mechanisms of support, an institute's budget is arranged by program areas and activities. Within these areas,

TABLE 3.2. Labor, Health and Human Services,
Education and Related Agencies Subcommittee
of the Senate Committee on Appropriations

Majority Members	Minority Members
Tom Harkin, IA (Chairman)	Arlen Specter, PA (Ranking)
Robert Byrd, WV	Mark Hatfield, OR
Ernest Hollings, SC	Ted Stevens, AK
Quentin Burdick, ND	Warren Rudman, NH
Daniel Inouye, HI	Thad Cochran, MS
Dale Bumpers, AR	Phil Gramm, TX
Harry Reid, NV	Slade Gorton, WA
Brock Adams, WA	

TABLE 3.3. FY 1991 NIH Budget

Extramural	Number	%	Award ($1,000)	%
Research Project Grants (RPG)*				
Noncompeting	15,401	71.2	3,296,869	73.3
Administrative supplement	440	2.0	20,642	0.5
Competing	5,785	26.8	1,180,122	26.2
Total	21,626		4,497,633	
Centers				
Noncompeting	515	76.6	545,393	76.4
Competing	157	23.4	168,102	23.6
Total	672		713,495	
Career (K)				
Noncompeting	1,231	77.2	90,123	76.7
Competing	364	22.8	27,333	23.3
Total	1,595		117,456	
Other (BRSG, MBRS, etc.)				
Noncompeting	1,106	42.5	176,498	62.8
Competing	1,495	57.5	104,391	37.2
Total	2,601		280,889	
Research and Development Contracts				
Renewal	1,220	91.7	555,967	90.4
New	111	8.3	59,069	9.6
Total	1,331		615,036	
Cancer control				
Total	252		68,789	
Construction				
Total			6,800	
National Library of Medicine				
Total			25,491	

Research Training	Number of Trainees/ Training Positions	%	Award ($1,000)	%
Individual				
Noncompeting	995	52.4	27,893	53.4
Competing	905	47.6	24,361	46.6
Total	1,900		52,254	
Institutional				
Noncompeting	8,741	85.0	219,315	86.3
Competing	1,537	15.0	34,817	13.7
Total	10,278		254,132	
Total Extramural			6,631,975	

(*continued*)

TABLE 3.3. (*Continued*)

Intramural	924,921
Research management and support	370,688
Cancer control (intramural)	16,900
National Library of Medicine	65,917
Office of the Director	97,651
Buildings and facilties	168,687
Total NIH	8,276,739

*Includes P01, R01, R22, R29, R35, R37, R43, R44, and U01

allotments are made for the various mechanisms of support. In a typical institute such as the NHLBI, the program areas and activities are:

- Heart and vascular diseases
- Lung diseases
- Blood diseases and resources
- Construction
- Intramural research
- National Research Service Awards (training)
- Research management and support

In addition to these allocated funds, the OD/NIH has discretionary funds to enhance program priorities and satisfy special needs of the NIH.

To move funds from one line item to another, an institute must forward a reprogramming request to the director of the NIH. The request usually is granted, unless the amount is more than $250,000 or 5 percent of the budgeted item, whichever is greater. Permission is usually denied if the program area from which the funds are taken is of special interest to the NIH or Congress. Permission to reprogram is required from Congress when funds are sequestered, e.g., when the rules mandated by the Gramm-Rudman-Hollings legislation are invoked. Also, congressional permission depends on the amounts to be moved and the sensitivity of the issue. Starting new programs and activities or changing or abolishing established ones must be approved by Congress.

Comparative appropriation figures for the fiscal years 1981–91 are presented in Table 3.4. Several NIH divisions and centers are not appropriated funds directly. Thus, for example, the Clinical Center and the Division of Research Grants (DRG) are supported by a management fund controlled by the Office of the Director. This fund is made up of a surtax imposed on each institute's appropriation. For example, DRG's share is based on the number of applications processed and reviewed in the previous year.

Thus, the general process is one in which the budget requests are developed by

TABLE 3.4. NIH Appropriations by NIH Component, Fiscal Years 1981–91
(Dollars in Thousands)

NIH Component	1981	1982	1983	1984	1985	1986
Total	$3,569,406	$3,641,875	$4,023,969	$4,476,141	$5,144,650	$5,494,398
NIA	75,608	81,903	93,996	114,921	144,444	156,352
NIAID	232,077	235,895	279,129	314,117	370,779	383,231
NIADDK	369,462	368,191	413,492	462,578	542,937	568,724
NIAMS	—	—	—	—	—	—
NCI	989,355	986,617	987,642	1,077,303	1,181,949	1,256,147
NICHD	220,628	226,309	254,324	275,179	313,150	321,581
NIDCD	—	—	—	—	—	—
NIDR	71,114	71,983	79,292	88,163	100,633	103,207
NIDDK	—	—	—	—	—	—
NIEHS	93,491	106,270	164,867	179,806	194,553	197,379
NEI	117,983	127,374	141,901	154,683	181,586	194,993
NIGMS	333,764	339,862	369,813	415,644	482,168	514,528
NHLBI	549,693	559,637	624,259	703,197	804,456	858,570
NINCDS	252,533	265,901	297,064	335,205	396,683	433,094
NINDS	—	—	—	—	—	—
DRR/NCRR	175,627	184,177	213,917	242,636	303,854	305,553
FIC	9,124	9,205	10,147	11,336	11,578	11,390
NCHGR	—	—	—	—	—	—
NCNR	—	—	—	—	—	—
NLM	44,666	45,035	51,943	49,613	55,848	57,759
OD	22,531	23,618	24,683	26,720	38,302	116,990**
Buildings and facilities	11,750	9,898	17,500	25,040	21,730	14,900

the authorized components within NIH, refined in terms of funding levels and policy in the OD, and sent to the USPHS, OASH, DHHS, and OMB, where each in turn provides its input. The President presents the budget to Congress, which holds hearings and enacts authorization and appropriation legislation. The OMB then releases the funds to the agency.

Table 3.5 and Figures 3.1 and 3.2 demonstrate the remarkable growth of NIH extramural grant and contract awards over a ten-year period.

Committees hearing testimony for authorization of NIH programs are the Health and Environment subcommittee of the Committee on Energy and Commerce of the House of Representatives and the Committee on Labor and Human Resources of the Senate (Tables 3.6 and 3.7). Information on authorizations, appropriations,

Table 3.4. (*Continued*)

| 1987* | 1988 | 1989† | 1990‡ | 1991 | Percentage change | |
					1981–91	1990–91
$6,180,660	$6,666,693	$7,152,207	$7,576,352	$8,276,739	131.9%	9.2%
176,931	194,746	222,643	239,455	323,752	328.2	35.2
545,523	638,800	744,152	832,977	906,251	290.5	8.8
—	—	—	—	—	—	—
138,713	147,679	159,897	168,930	193,247	—	14.4
1,402,837	1,469,327	1,571,879	1,634,332	1,714,784	73.3	4.9
366,780	396,811	425,649	442,914	478,956	117.1	8.1
—	—	91,677	117,583	134,935	—	14.8
117,945	126,297	130,752	135,749	148,918	109.4	9.7
511,124	534,733	559,538	581,477	615,272	—	5.8
209,294	215,666	223,454	229,234	241,028	157.8	5.1
216,637	224,947	231,230	236,533	253,241	114.6	7.1
570,916	632,676	682,349	681,782	760,010	127.7	11.5
930,001	965,536	1,045,985	1,072,354	1,126,942	105.0	5.1
490,233	534,692	—	—	—	—	—
—	—	474,943	490,409	541,743	—	10.5
322,860	368,153	358,608	353,734	335,255	90.9	−5.2
11,420	15,651	15,848	15,516	17,519	92.0	12.9
—	—	—	59,538	87,418	—	46.8
19,000	23,380	29,139	33,513	39,722	—	18.5
61,838	67,910	73,731	81,861	91,408	104.6	11.7
56,708	61,819	72,201	107,419	97,651	333.4	−9.1
31,900	47,870	38,532	61,042	168,687	1,335.6	176.3

*In 1987, NIAMS, NIDDK, and NCNR appropriations were new.

†In 1989, NIDCD and NINDS appropriations were new.

‡In 1990, NCHGR appropriation was new, and DRR was reorganized and renamed NCRR.

**Includes AIDS funds appropriated to OD but transferred out to be awarded and administered. Also includes funds for NCNR which were administered under OD in 1986.

(From the Office of Science Policy and Legislation, National Institutes of Health. 1991. *NIH data book*. Bethesda, Md.)

and other legislative matters, including testimonies before congressional committees, can be obtained from:

Division of Legislative Analysis
Building 1, Room 244
NIH
Bethesda, MD 20892
(301) 496–3471

TABLE 3.5. NIH Awards by Funding Mechanism, Fiscal Years 1981–90 (Dollars in Millions)

Funding mechanism	1981	1982	1983	1984	1985	1986	1987	1988	1989	1990
Amount										
Total	$2,883.7	$2,930.1	$3,246.4	$3,657.6	$4,248.1	$4,426.6	$5,194.2	$5,544.8	$6,009.0	$6,281.8
R&D grants	2,331.4	2,407.7	2,702.3	3,087.0	3,591.3	3,739.1	4,401.2	4,727.3	5,054.7	5,239.8
R&D contracts	366.9	358.7	370.3	394.7	417.7	462.6	544.4	565.1	657.2	714.9
Research training	181.7	156.3	171.1	173.2	224.0	217.1	238.8	245.7	261.0	292.2
Individual awards	35.5	31.2	34.4	34.4	46.4	42.8	46.6	45.0	45.9	50.9
Institutional awards	146.2	125.1	136.7	138.8	177.5	174.4	192.1	200.6	215.1	241.4
Construction grants	2.0	6.2	1.5	1.0	12.1	5.0	6.9	—	—	14.8
Grants for repair, renovation, and modernization of existing research facilities								—	28.9	11.0
Other	1.6	1.1	1.2	1.7	3.0	2.8	3.0	6.7	7.2	9.0
Number										
R&D grants	20,418	19,893	20,819	21,535	22,958	23,445	25,026	25,754	26,022	25,725
R&D contracts	1,340	1,180	1,110	1,150	1,335	1,298	1,257	1,252	1,311	1,332
Research training	3,121	3,020	3,096	3,119	3,341	3,157	3,404	3,348	3,277	3,863
Individual awards	1,752	1,726	1,756	1,759	1,985	1,823	2,032	1,944	1,845	2,406
Institutional awards	1,369	1,294	1,340	1,360	1,356	1,334	1,372	1,404	1,432	1,457
Construction grants	6	18	3	3	33	29	35	—	—	7

(From the Office of Science Policy and Legislation, National Institutes of Health. 1991. *NIH data book*. Bethesda, Md.)

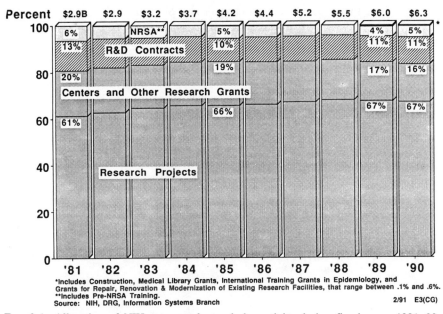

FIG. 3.1. Allocation of NIH extramural awards by activity during fiscal years 1981–90 (percent of amount awarded). (From the Division of Research Grants, National Institutes of Health. 1991. *Extramural Trends*. Bethesda, Md.)

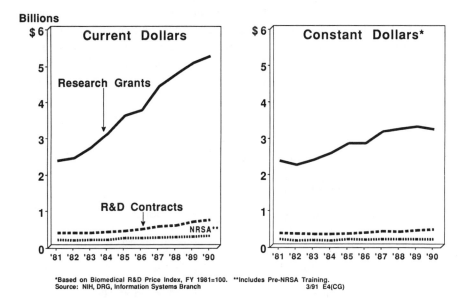

FIG. 3.2. NIH extramural awards by activity during fiscal years 1981–90. (From the Division of Research Grants, National Institutes of Health. 1991. *Extramural Trends*. Bethesda, Md.)

TABLE 3.6. Health and Environment Subcommittee of the House Committee on Energy and Commerce, 102nd Congress

Majority Members	Minority Members
Henry Waxman, CA (Chairman)	William Dannemeyer, CA (Ranking)
Gerry Sikorski, KS	Thomas Bliley, Jr., VA
Terry Bruce, IL	Jack Fields, TX
J. Roy Rowland, GA	Michael Bilirakis, FL
Edolphus Towns, NY	Alex McMillan, NC
Gerry Studds, MA	J. Dennis Hastert, IL
Peter Kostmayer, PA	Clyde Holloway, LA
James Scheuer, NY	
Mike Synar, OK	
Ron Wyden, OR	
Ralph Hall, TX	
Bill Richardson, NM	
John Bryant, TX	

MANAGING THE COSTS OF BIOMEDICAL RESEARCH

While Congress has always thought that it was generous in funding the NIH, it was concerned over the many calls and letters from members of the research community about the NIH budget and the "funding crisis." Following an analysis of factors contributing to this crisis, the House Appropriations Subcommittee made a number of suggestions about approaches to funding, most of which were adopted by NIH, in whole or in part. NIH has put into effect the following approaches to managing costs.

TABLE 3.7. Senate Committee on Labor and Human Resources, 102nd Congress

Majority Members	Minority Members
Edward Kennedy, MA (Chairman)	Orrin Hatch, UT (Ranking)
Claiborne Pell, RI	Nancy Kassebaum, KS
Howard Metzenbaum, OH	James Jeffords, VT
Christopher Dodd, CT	Dan Coats, IN
Paul Simon, IL	Strom Thurmond, SC
Tom Harkin, IA	Dave Durenberger, MN
Brock Adams, WA	Thad Cochran, MS
Barbara Mikulski, MD	
Jeff Bingaman, NM	
Paul Wellstone, MN	

Starting with FY 1991 competing awards, the average duration of a grant was set at four years (the average had risen from 3.0 to 4.2 years during the 1980s). This will still allow for five-year awards; however, fewer such grants are likely to be made in the future.

NIH eliminated across-the-board reductions of the budget after the first year of the competitive segment of the grant.

In future years of grant support, growth of the costs of projects will not exceed an average of 4 percent.

A triage step was set up in which the bottom third of all applications given priority ratings routinely will not be considered by advisory councils. Although not all ICDs observe this practice rigidly, there will be a tendency for fewer applications to be considered by the councils for funding.

To enable councils to consider total costs (direct plus indirect) of proposed projects, total costs requested and recommended are now included on summary statements.

NIH uses the first-year indirect cost rate throughout all years of the grant.

Reviewers are instructed to scrutinize proposed budgets more closely.

PRIVACY ACT (PA) AND FREEDOM OF INFORMATION ACT (FOIA)

Legislation enacted in 1974 provides access to government files by the public. The PA permits individuals to:

- Determine what records pertaining to them are maintained in a federal agency
- Prevent their records from being used for any purpose other than the intended one(s) without their permission
- Gain access to and examine their records
- Ascertain that the information concerning them is accurate

The term "record" refers to any item of information about an individual that is contained in an agency system of records or files and is retrievable by the individual's name. An example at NIH would be the grant files kept in an institute or study section office. Further information regarding the PA and its implications for PIs and applicants can be obtained from:

NIH Privacy Act Officer
Division of Management Policy
Building 31, Room 3B07
NIH
Bethesda, MD 20892
(301) 496–2832

The FOIA provides for a third party to gain information from records held by the federal government. If an individual or an organization wants information from records other than their own, the FOIA applies. In the case of NIH extramural programs, the FOIA applies to funded new grants (Type 1), competing continuation (Type 2), noncompeting continuation (Type 5), and supplemental (Type 3) applications. There are a number of exemptions to disclosure, but three especially relate to NIH:

- Trade secrets, commercial and financial information
- Inter- or intra-agency memoranda or letters that would be available only by litigation
- Records whose release would constitute an unwarranted invasion of privacy

Under these exemptions, for example, summary statements are not released to persons other than the principal investigator (PI). Also, if a FOIA request is made, the PI has the right to request deletion from the application of information concerning the three areas above. Additional information can be obtained from the particular ICD Freedom of Information coordinator or:

NIH Freedom of Information Officer
Building 1, Room 344
NIH
Bethesda, MD 20892
(301) 496–4461

GOVERNMENT IN THE SUNSHINE ACT

This 1976 legislation is intended to open to the public as many meetings of federal agencies as possible. Thus, at least part of all NIH public advisory committee (study sections and advisory councils) meetings must be open. However, only the portion dealing with administrative, programmatic, and policy matters is open. Any part related to the review of grant applications is closed.

FEDERAL ADVISORY COMMITTEE ACT

This legislation requires notices of meetings of advisory committees be published in the *Federal Register*. These notices must appear, at a minimum, fifteen days before the meeting. The Act also spells out conditions of membership on review committees. Additional information can be obtained from:

NIH Committee Management Office
Building 1, Room B1–56
NIH
Bethesda, MD 20892
(301) 496–2123

4

Extramural Support Mechanisms

A substantial array of extramural support mechanisms is available covering every stage of the research career spectrum. An overview is provided in this chapter and a brief summary of the various mechanisms included in Appendix 2, along with FY 1991 success rates and average costs per award. There are three major categories of awards, detailed below.

RESEARCH GRANTS

Research grants, the largest category, includes awards for a variety of research projects and research training activities. The important features of a grant are:

- The idea for the research or training project is initiated by the investigator and not by the NIH. In the case of Requests for Applications (RFAs), the NIH identifies the general objective of the solicitation and depends on the creative talent of the principal investigator (PI) to provide the approaches and methodology.
- Freedom to pursue the research without NIH staff involvement
- No expectation on the part of NIH for delivery of a specific product
- Duration of time usually no more than five years

RESEARCH AND DEVELOPMENT (R AND D) CONTRACTS

Contracts are used to satisfy specialized institute R and D needs under the following conditions:

- Specific research problem identified by NIH
- Concept undergoes peer review by an advisory committee before issuance of an RFP

- Individual proposals peer reviewed by a scientific review group
- NIH staff monitoring to ensure objectives/product "deliverables" are met
- Expectation that the research or development goals will be accomplished and made available to the NIH

COOPERATIVE AGREEMENTS

Cooperative agreements such as those described below are being used with greater frequency when cooperation between NIH and investigators is indicated.

- Idea initiated by the NIH
- Concept undergoes peer review by an advisory committee before issuance of an RFA
- Substantial programmatic involvement by NIH staff, which must be defined in the RFA
- Collaborative type of arrangement with NIH, e.g., clinical trial
- Policies, application procedures, and the review process similar to those for R01s or related types of grant mechanisms

The key features of each type of major award category are highlighted in Table 4.1.

In the vast majority of cases, unsolicited, investigator-initiated grant requests predominate. However, the NIH does employ techniques to stimulate submission of research grant applications and cooperative agreements in areas of special program interest. The two most well-known methods are the use of program announcements and requests for applications.

PROGRAM ANNOUNCEMENTS (PA)

PAs describes a special area of new or ongoing program interest that an ICD may wish to stimulate or expand. These also can be used to announce a new mechanism of grant support.

TABLE 4.1. Features of Major NIH Award Categories

Mechanism	NIH Role
Grant	Patron (encouragement, assistance but no staff involvement)
Contract	Purchaser (procurement instrument)
Cooperative Agreement	Partner (assistance but substantial staff involvement)

- Program announcements appear in the *NIH Guide for Grants and Contracts.*
- Interest is not limited to a specific time period even though announcement may appear only once.
- Applications can be submitted to meet any of the deadline dates for regular research grants.
- Applications are treated in the same way as regular research grants and are peer reviewed by DRG study sections.
- There are no funds set aside for these applications.

REQUEST FOR APPLICATIONS (RFA)

An RFA solicits grant applications in a well-defined scientific area corresponding to a special program initiative identified by an ICD's staff, program advisory committee, or advisory council.

- Announcements appear in the *NIH Guide for Grants and Contracts.*
- This is a one-time competition.
- The deadline date is specified in the RFA.
- Applications received are peer reviewed as a group, usually by an institute ad hoc review committee.
- Funds are set aside for each RFA competition.

While a host of support mechanisms currently exists, new ones are constantly being generated. New extramural support mechanisms can originate in several ways. The Congress can specifically direct that programs and mechanisms be initiated. There are numerous examples, including the Specialized Centers of Research (SCOR) programs and the Comprehensive Centers in the NHLBI. The 1 percent set aside for the SBIR (R23 and R24) program was imposed on the NIH and other agencies by Congress. Another route is special interest foundations and other groups within the scientific community which may identify a need and transmit it via program advisory committees, national advisory councils, or workshops. Finally, the NIH staff may recognize a particular need not sufficiently addressed by existing mechanisms. A prime example has been the desire to encourage more physicians to pursue research careers, resulting in the Physician Scientist Awards (PSA) (K11, K12, K15, K16) as well as the Clinical Investigator Award (CIA) (K08). The desire to promote greater support stability for investigators led to the Outstanding Investigator (R35) and MERIT Award (R37) programs. The concern to ensure adequate support for new investigators gave birth eventually to the First Independent Research Support and Transition Award (FIRST) (R29) (successor to the NIRA [R23] award). The numerous new mechanisms, expanded use of RFAs, including cooperative agreements, and the past trend toward longer awards, have all contributed to the enormous pressures that currently exists on the research grant portion of the NIH extramural budget.

TABLE 4.2. FY 1991 Data on NIH Competing Grant Applications

	Number			Success*
Mechanism	Reviewed	Eligible[†]	Awarded	Rate (%)
Research project grant (RPG) applications—totals	19,501	18,635	5,770	29.6
Traditional (R01)	15,047	14,797	4,174	27.7
New	10,357	10,080	2,227	21.5
Competing continuation	4,640	4,667	1,919	41.4
Supplements (competing)	50	50	28	56.0
Program project (P01)	407	400	207	50.9
New	191	187	74	38.7
Competing continuation	165	164	106	64.2
Supplements (competing)	51	49	27	52.9
R22 (U.S./Japan program)	48	48	13	27.1
First (R29)	1,445	1,438	450	31.1
OIG (R35)	18	21	9	50.0
Merit (R37)	245	253	239	97.6
SBIR (R43)	1,611	1,082	428	26.6
SBIR (R44)	291	241	126	43.3
U01 (Cooperative agreement)	389	355	125	32.1
Research centers—totals	446	426	209	46.9
GCRC (M01)	59	57	42	71.2
Exploratory/planning (P20)	35	31	16	45.7
Core (P30)	160	156	66	41.3
Animal resource (P40)	9	8	3	33.3
Biotechnical resource (P41)	28	28	13	46.4
Specialized (P50)	85	83	39	45.9
Primate (P51)	14	14	13	92.9
Comprehensive (P60)	44	37	6	13.6
RCMIs (G12)	12	12	11	91.7
Research career development awards—totals	598	556	298	49.8
RCDA (K04)	93	87	40	43.0
Adademic/teacher (K07)	91	82	36	39.6
CIA (K08)	270	248	143	53.0
PSA (K11)	135	131	73	54.1
DSA (K15)	9	8	6	66.7

(continued)

TABLE 4.2. (*Continued*)

| Mechanism | Number | | | Success* |
	Reviewed	Eligible†	Awarded	Rate (%)
Program—totals	11	11	9	81.8
PSA (K12)	2	3	3	100.0
DSA (K16)	9	8	6	66.7
Research training awards—totals	2401	2316	1203	50.1
Individual predoctoral (F31)	261	247	198	75.9
Individual postdoctoral (F32)	1,697	1,624	730	43.0
Senior fellowship (F33)	44	41	22	50.0
Institutional (T32)	399	404	253	63.4
Other grant programs—totals	1757	1583	506	28.2
Small grant (R03)	849	727	156	18.4
Conference (R13)	295	282	211	71.5
AREA (R15)	613	574	139	22.7

Source: ISB, DRG

*Success rate equals number funded/number reviewed.

†Includes a small number of applications carried over from the prior fiscal year. In the case of the Research Project Grant category, this represents 148 or 0.8 percent of the 18,635 applications. A similar situation obtains for several of the other mechanisms listed.

To provide greater insight about NIH grant awards, Tables 4.2, 4.3, 4.4, and 4.5 indicate: the number of competitive applications received and processed in FY 1991 for the more prominent mechanisms; the chances for success; the R01 funding record of the institutes; and data on amended applications.

The category "Research Project Grant Applications" (RPG) is commonly used in several DRG publications describing data about the extramural programs. This category is a mixture, made up of several types of research grant mechanisms identified in Table 4.2.

What about amended applications? Is it worthwhile to reapply? The data for FY 1990 indicate the answer to be affirmative. Considering *only R01* applications reviewed by DRG study sections (R01-type applications received in response to RFAs are usually reviewed by ICD committees):

- 34.4 percent of competing applications were amendments.
- 31.3 percent of new applications were amendments.
- 41.0 percent of competing continuations were amendments.
- 38.2 percent of the awards for new and competing continuations were amended applications.

The data for FY 1990 for RPGs which is a *mixture of mechanisms* identified in Table 4.2, provides more insight into the number and award rates of amended applica-

TABLE 4.3. FY 1991 Institute Success Rates for Several
Prominent Mechanisms

Institute	Mechanism				
	P01	R01	R29	F32	T32
NCI	44.0	24.4	34.2	33.8	62.5
NHLBI	49.0	23.9	32.2	56.6	55.0
NIDR	41.7	30.1	41.9	72.7	23.1
NIDDK	46.9	24.2	28.9	48.9	47.6
NINDS	67.6	29.5	28.1	48.6	60.0
NIAID	38.7	28.2	37.0	36.6	78.9
NIGMS	59.1	34.6	28.6	33.6	94.1
NICHD	51.6	25.2	21.1	49.5	77.1
NEI	—	32.8	28.6	56.4	44.4
NIEHS	66.7	25.7	33.3	66.7	50.0
NIA	63.5	29.0	23.6	59.3	81.3
NIAMS	30.0	31.3	42.3	37.8	77.8
NCNR	—	24.7	11.1	16.7	00.0
NIDCD	50.0	28.9	42.2	69.7	85.7
NCHGR	60.0	38.3	00.0	36.4	25.0
NCRR	—	20.5	00.0	00.0	100.0
Overall percentage	50.9	27.7	31.1	43.0	63.4

Source: ISB, DRG

tions. In 1980, there were 2,200 amended applications, which grew to 6,300 in
1990. The percentages of amended applications and the award rates for three past
fiscal years are included in Table 4.5.

What are some of the other characteristics of the RPG program for FY 1990?

The traditional research project (R01) grant mechanism has always been considered
the mainstay of the grant programs. It is an award made to support the research,
usually of a single investigator, on a fairly focused subject. In FY 1990, about
57 percent of the grant applications received by the NIH fell into the R01
category.

The average length of RPG awards was 4.2 years in contrast to 3.3 years in 1983.
This has caused an increase in the noncompeting NIH grant budget (commitment base) and is one reason for the declining award rates. The new NIH target
is to maintain an average award rate of 4.0 years (see Chapter 3).

Noncompeting continuations accounted for 77 percent of the NIH RPG budget,
competing continuations 11 percent, new applications 11 percent, and supplements 1 percent (see Table 3.3, Chapter 3, for FY 1991 data).

TABLE 4.4. FY 1991 Institute Success Rates for Types of R01 Applications

ICD	Overall Rate (%)	New Applications			Renewals			Supplements		
		REV	AWD	%	REV	AWD	%	REV	AWD	%
NCI	24.4	1,606	329	20.5	710	235	33.1	4	1	25.0
NHLBI	23.9	1,434	255	17.8	572	222	38.8	9	5	55.6
NIDR	30.1	219	51	23.3	100	45	45.0	—	—	—
NIDDK	24.2	1,051	186	17.7	512	191	37.3	4	2	50.0
NINDS	29.5	834	187	22.4	457	191	41.8	9	5	55.6
NIAID	28.2	989	237	24.0	383	149	38.9	—	1	—
NIGMS	34.6	1,237	283	22.9	819	428	52.3	2	2	100.0
NICHD	25.2	784	154	19.6	364	134	36.8	7	3	42.9
NEI	32.8	343	85	24.8	274	118	43.1	1	0	00.0
NIEHS	25.7	220	48	21.8	93	31	33.3	2	2	100.0
NIA	29.0	673	173	25.7	110	55	50.0	2	0	00.0
NIAMS	31.3	374	100	26.7	135	60	44.4	2	0	00.0
NCNR	24.7	145	32	22.1	20	8	40.0	1	1	100.0
NIDCD	28.9	224	41	18.3	76	42	55.3	4	5	100.0
NCHGR	38.3	139	51	36.7	12	7	58.3	3	1	33.3
NCRR	20.5	85	15	17.6	3	3	100.0	—	—	—
Totals	27.7*	10,357	2,227	21.5*	4,640	1,919	41.4*	50	28	56.0*

*Averages.
Abbreviations: REV = reviewed; AWD = awarded.
Source: ISB; DRG.

Five-year requests have increased from 22 to 52 percent from FY 1983 to FY 1990. Three-year requests have declined in that same period from 63 to 32 percent.

Indirect cost rates have increased from 28.6 percent in FY 1980 to 31.7 percent in FY 1990 of the NIH research grant budget.

Distribution of direct costs on approved budgets was: personnel 65.1 percent; equipment 4.3 percent; supplies 12.4 percent; and all other expenses 18.2 percent.

Fifty-two percent of the NIH research grant budget was used to fund competing and

TABLE 4.5. Data on Amended RPG Applications

FY	Percentage of Applications			Percentage of Awards		
	Total	New	Renewal	Total	New	Renewal
1980	15.4	14.8	17.3	12.2	13.3	10.5
1985	22.0	20.8	25.7	22.6	23.5	21.3
1990	29.4	27.0	36.1	34.1	36.2	31.1

non-competing R01s. Three ICDs awarded more than 70 percent of their research grant budget to R01s: NEI (76 percent), NIGMS (75 percent), and NCNR (70 percent).

EXAMPLES OF THE USE OF MECHANISMS AT VARIOUS CAREER STAGES

Health Professional Degree (D.D.S., M.D., D.O., D.V.M., or equivalent)

Career Stage

Health Professional School. Students can seek appointment to a T35 (Short-Term Training for Students in Health Professional Schools) grant, if one is available at the institution, or appointment to other types of grants, e.g., R01, P01

Clinical Training: There are no mechanisms to support strictly clinical/residency training.

Postclinical: The Physician Scientist Program (K11 and K12 for M.D.s; K15 and K16 for D.D.S.s) is designed to train clinicians, with little or no research experience, for careers as independent investigators. During phase II, the last three years of the five-year program, one is eligible to apply for a FIRST award. The sequence can continue with R01 support, overlapping K04 support, and, at an appropriate time, K07 support. The National Research Service Award (NRSA) Senior Fellowship (F33) program or Fogarty Center International Fellowships are available if midcareer adjustments are desirable.

Another option is to begin research training with an NRSA Individual Postdoctoral Fellowship (F32) or appointment to a similar position in a T32 (NRSA Institutional Training Grant) program, if one is available at the institution. This can be followed with a Clinical Investigator Award (K08). After an award is made, application may be made for a FIRST award. The sequence can continue with R01 support, overlapping K04 support, and, at an appropriate time, K07 support. The F33 (NRSA Senior Fellowship) program or Fogarty Center International Fellowships are available if midcareer adjustments are desirable.

NIH staff should be consulted about eligibility requirements, availability of mechanisms, and other award options.

Graduate Degree (Ph.D. or equivalent)

Career Stage

Graduate Student. Support can be obtained by appointment to an NRSA Institutional Training Grant (T32) or by serving as a research assistant on an R01 or other types of research grants.

Postdoctoral. Support can be obtained from an NRSA Individual Postdoctoral Fellowship (F32) or by appointment to a T32 program, if one is available at the institution.

Independent Investigator. One can start by applying for a FIRST award. The sequence can continue with R01 support, overlapping K04 support, and, at an appropriate time, K07 support. The F33 (NRSA Senior Fellowship) program or Fogarty Center International Fellowships are available if midcareer adjustments are desirable.

Special mention should be made of the K awards. There are several types available and sometimes it is difficult to distinguish among them. Appendix 2 provides assistance in this respect. Table 4.6 attempts to compare characteristics of three types of K awards.

NIH staff should be consulted about eligibility requirements, availability of mechanisms, and other award options.

TABLE 4.6. K Award Characteristics

Clinical Investigator Awards (K08)	Physician Scientist Award (K11)	Research Center Development Award (K04)
Purpose		
To prepare clinical investigators who have had some research experience for independent research careers	To prepare clinicians who have no or little research experience for independent research careers	To support further development of junior faculty by allowing maximum effort to be spent in research
Eligibility		
Clinical degree	Clinical degree	Research training complete
Clinical experience		
Normally have finished clinical training	May have had only one year of clinical training	N/A
Research experience		
Yes	Normally no; requires structured training program	Yes
Sponsor requirement		
Yes	Yes	No
Sponsor salary support		
No	Yes, for phase I of research training	N/A
Salary support		
Up to $50,000 plus fringe benefits	Up to $50,000 plus fringe benefits	Up to $50,000 plus fringe benefits

GENERAL COMMENTS

Members of the scientific community have relied heavily for their research support on the R01 program. Unfortunately, that support is dwindling and causing deep frustration and disappointment for those who have become accustomed to, and dependent upon, such support. Based on FY 1991 data, the chances of a new (Type 1) application resulting in an award are about 1 in 5. For competing continuations (renewals), the chances are about 1 in 2.5 that an application will result in an award.

What are the options for applicants? For new applicants that meet the criteria for the FIRST program, the chances for success are better (about 1 in 3) and the award provides five years of support. However, the disadvantages should be considered in that the award requires a 50 percent time commitment and provides a modest funding ceiling which may be insufficient, especially for clinical research. For the vast majority of investigators who have been nurtured on R01 support, perhaps the time is right to become more familiar with other NIH programs and support mechanisms. Several of the ICDs are more heavily invested in research grants than others. Several have above-average funding rates, e.g., NEI and NIGMS. If you are aware of their program interests, you might be surprised to learn that your research interests coincide. Get your name on the mailing list for the *NIH Guide for Grants and Contracts*. Read about the RFAs, the PAs, other solicitations, and new mechanisms of support. Work closely with your Office of Sponsored Research. Seek out colleagues who are familiar with the grant programs and obtain their advice. Is there potential for team research efforts and collaborations at your institution? The chances for obtaining P01 and center support may be worth exploring (see Tables 4.2 and 4.3). Also, depending on your career status, reviewing the various K awards may prove beneficial. Finally, Chapter 14 includes a variety of helpful sources of information.

EXTRAMURAL SUPPORT MECHANISMS FOR
UNDERREPRESENTED MINORITIES

NIH and Congress have recognized the need to enhance and strengthen the research and research training opportunities for minority groups. To this end and to assist minority institutions in improving their facilities and research potential, a number of programs have been developed. Support mechanisms directed at underrepresented minorities are numerous and varied. They cover the spectrum of education and career levels for individuals and focus on institutions of higher learning as well. The term "underrepresented minority" refers primarily to blacks, Hispanics, native Americans, Asian/Pacific Islanders, and Alaskan natives.

Appendix 3 briefly describes most of the award programs in this category. Success rates and total cost per award are included in Appendix 2. Only one program is detailed here because of its wide applicability to the most prominent grant programs.

All NIH awarding units are accepting requests for *administrative* supplements to ongoing research grants to encourage members of minority groups to participate in biomedical and behavioral research. Supplements to the following types of grants are acceptable: R01, R10 (clinical trial), R18 (demonstration activities), R24 (resource-related project), R35, R37, P01, P40, P41, P50, P60, or U01. A separate program announcement is available for each of three target groups: undergraduate students, graduate research assistants, and faculty members (*NIH Guide for Grants and Contracts*, Vol. 18, No. 14, April 21, 1989).

The programs for the three target groups have several features in common. The parent grants must be at domestic institutions and have at least two years of support remaining at time of any supplemental award. There are no deadline dates. Applications can be submitted at any time directly to the awarding unit. Notification of funding decisions is provided approximately four weeks from the date the application is submitted.

The following items are to be included in the application:

- Completed face page from PHS Form 398 application kit with parent grant title and number and which of the three types of supplements is being requested
- Brief description of parent grant and plans for involving minority individual (3–4 pages, prepared by PI)
- Statement from minority candidate outlining research and career goals
- Curriculum vitae of minority candidate including past scientific experience
- Proposed budget

Review criteria:

- Qualifications of minority candidate
- Plans for the proposed research experience
- Assurance from PI that minority candidate will be an integral part of the project and will benefit from the experience
- Others as specified in each program announcement

More specific information and detail are contained in the Program Announcement and briefly mentioned below:

Research Supplements for Minority Undergraduate Students

Description

This supplement provides funds to permit minority undergraduate students to obtain research experience for three months during the summer or at other times separate from an academic program.

Comments

As a means of identifying qualified undergraduate students, lists of participants in other related programs can be obtained from the NIH (Minority Access to Research Careers and Minority Biomedical Research Support programs). Students may be recruited either from the applicant institution or other institutions. They can be compensated at the rate of $6.00 per hour plus $125 per month for supplies and travel. Support is for three months of fulltime effort per year for a minimum of two years.

Awarding Units

All NIH awarding units.

Research Supplements for Minority Graduate Assistants

Description

This supplement provides funds to permit predoctoral students to enhance their research experience by participating in a funded research project.

ICD	Address	Telephone
NIA	Gateway Building, Room 2C218	(301) 496–9322
NIAID	Solar Building, Room 4C07	(301) 496–7291
NIAMS	Building 31, Room 4C32	(301) 496–0802
NICHD	Executive Plaza North, Room 520	(301) 496–1485
NCI	Westwood Building, Room 850	(301) 496–7173
NIDCD	Executive Plaza South, Room 400	(301) 496–1804
NIDR	Westwood Building, Room 510	(301) 496–6324
NIDDK	Westwood Building, Room 657	(301) 496–7277
NIEHS	Building 3, Room 305A P.O. Box 12233 Research Triangle Park, NC 27709	(919) 629–7634
NEI	Building 31, Room 6A48	(301) 496–5884
NIGMS	Westwood Building, Room 938	(301) 496–7061
NHLBI	Westwood Building, Room 7A17B	(301) 496–7416
NLM	Building 38A, Room 5N505	(301) 496–4621
NINDS	Federal Building, Room 1016A	(301) 496–9248
NCHGR	Building 38A, Room 612	(301) 496–7531
NCNR	Building 31, Room 5B03	(301) 496–0523
NCRR	Westwood Building, Room 10A14	(301) 496–9971
FIC	Building 31, Room B2C39	(301) 496–1653

All of the above addresses, with the NIEHS exception, end with NIH, Bethesda, MD 20892.

Comments

Awards are limited to minority predoctoral students actively pursuing a degree in the biomedical or behavioral sciences at the applicant institution. Funds can be requested for salary commensurate with the institutional scale, as well as necessary expenses related to the project.

Awarding Units

All NIH awarding units.

Research Supplements for Minority Investigators

Description

This supplement provides funds to permit minority faculty members to enhance their research skills. There are two types.

Short-Term Supplements. These awards allow research to be conducted for 3–5 months per year, full-time during the summer, or at other times, for a minimum of two years and a maximum of four years.

Long-Term Supplements. These awards allow research to be conducted at a minimum of 30 percent effort per year for not less than two or more than four years.

Comments

Eligible investigators must have a doctoral degree, at least one year of postdoctoral experience, and be a faculty member at either the applicant or other institutions. Faculty members who served as PIs on previously funded R, K, or P series awards are ineligible. The exceptions are R03, R15, MBRS, and MARC awards. Awards are for a maximum of $50,000 (direct costs) per year with no more than $40,000 allocated for salary and fringe benefits. The balance can be used for supplies and travel, but not for equipment.

Awarding Units

All NIH awarding units.

The accompanying chart (p. 42) provides contacts for more information related to extramural support mechanisms.

5

Application Preparation

To enter the competitive fray for obtaining research grant funds, it is necessary for the investigator to transfer research ideas to paper. While there are a number of different application forms, the most common one is the PHS Form 398. Application kits are available at most applicant institutions, usually in the Office of Grants and Contracts or the Office of Sponsored Research. They also can be obtained from the Office of Grants Inquiries, DRG. The application forms used by the USPHS granting agencies are as follows:

- PHS 398; New, Competing Continuation, and Supplemental Research Project Grants, AREA Grants, FIRST Awards, Cooperative Agreements, Program Projects, Centers, RCDA, and National Research Service Institutional Awards
- PHS 6246–1; SBIR Program, Phase I
- PHS 6246–2; SBIR, Phase II
- PHS 416–1; Individual NRSA or Senior International Fellowship Award
- NIH 1541–1; International Research Fellowship Award
- PHS 6025; Nonresearch Training Grant
- PHS 5161–1; Grant to State or Local Government Agency; Health Services Project
- NIH 2575; Construction Grant
- NIH 147–1; Biomedical Research Support Grant
- NIH 1887; Medical Library Resource Improvement Grant

In this chapter, emphasis is on the PHS 398 for the Research Project (R01) Award, the FIRST (R29) Award, and the RCDA (K04); the PHS 416–1 for the Individual (F32) and Senior (F33) NRSA; and the PHS 6246–1 (R43) and -2 (R44) for the SBIR program.

To start, the following general advice is offered:

Submit a well-organized application; this indicates that the proposed research has been carefully planned.

Avoid a late submission. Plan ahead and get started early; have the final version ready well in advance of the appropriate receipt date.

Ease the way by reading the relevant NIH brochures and program announcements, e.g., "Helpful Hints" (Division of Research Grants, National Institutes of Health. 1990. *Helpful Hints on Preparing a Research Grant Application to the National Institutes of Health*. Bethesda, MD.), the "NIH Guide for Grants and Contracts", etc. Information on these publications is available from the Office of Grants Inquiries, DRG.

Do not hesitate to talk with appropriate NIH program and review staff. They cannot participate in writing the application or advise on what experiments to carry out, but they can provide information on application format, program interests, and policies and procedures. NIH staff contacts are included in Chapter 4 and chapters that follow. Awarding components of the USPHS with telephone numbers of staff contacts are also listed in Appendix 1.

Take advantage of the experience and knowledge of scientists and administrators at your own institutions. Offices of Sponsored Research and departmental business offices can offer invaluable advice.

If you are entering a new field or proposing a project somewhat peripheral to your usual area of work, be sure to provide the information and documentation that will convince the reviewers that you can accomplish what you propose to do.

Always use the most up-to-date application kit.

Read and follow the instructions; this is essential!

If your application is an amended (revised) version of a previously submitted but unfunded proposal, consider carefully the prospect of success and whether it is indeed worth trying again with this particular approach or project.

Be aware of the review criteria.

Try to determine the study section that will most likely review your proposal. The Referral Office of DRG can help you here (see Chapter 6). Then obtain a roster of its members from the latest copy of *NIH Advisory Committees* or from the study section office.

Approach the science of your project from a mechanistic point of view. Avoid an application that deals with phenomenological or observational research. The design of the experiments may be elegant, but the reviewers might view this approach as a non-innovative, descriptive or data-gathering exercise.

Senior investigators should not depend on their past records of accomplishment and a hastily prepared application for a favorable review. There is no substitute for a well-written application with clearly focused and well-designed experiments that go far in answering important and relevant research questions.

In making the most persuasive case for supporting your ideas, try to be aware of how your proposal will be received by the reviewers. Establish your research priorities. Be careful not to omit relevant information. Do not take anything for granted. You may think the reviewers know what you are getting at, but they want to know if *you* do.

Observe the page limitation rules. The type on the face page must be 10 characters per inch to assure computer processing of the data. The remainder of the application must consist of type of standard size, ten to twelve points (no more than fifteen characters per inch). There must not be more than six lines of text within a vertical inch. DRG will return applications that violate these stipulations.

The typing of the application should be legible. Avoid poor quality dot matrix printers, as the print may reproduce poorly.

Computer-generated facsimiles of the application form may be used, provided they maintain the exact wording and format of the government-printed forms, including all captions and spacing.

Proofread carefully. NIH will print and distribute approximately fifty copies of the application to staff, members of review panels, and advisory councils. Prepare the document as carefully as you would a research paper submitted to a journal.

In common usage, the terms "applicant" and "principal investigator" (PI) often are used interchangeably. However, officially, the institution is the applicant. The PI, an employee of the institution, is not. Remember, you are submitting an application and acting in the name of your organization.

PHS 398

For the preparation of applications, especially the traditional research project (R01), the following points are important:

Face Page

The institution, not NIH, determines who can be a PI on a grant application. One person should be named who will be responsible to the applicant institution for the scientific and technical direction of the project. While many projects are carried out by more than one principal participant, the concept of co-principal investigator is not formally recognized by the PHS.

Academic and professional degrees are important. NIH collects and reports this information to the research community and to Congress.

Choose a simple but relevant title with obvious health-related implications. Do not use an esoteric and confusing title. This can be taken out of context by individuals seeking to show that public funds are being sought by the research community to carry out what they consider to be "useless" projects.

Competing continuation and revised applications generally should have the same title as the original grant or application. However, if aims or directions have changed, a new title is acceptable. Supplemental applications must have the same title as the currently funded grant.

The relevant NIH computer program dictates that you stay within fifty-six spaces for the title or it will be changed by DRG.

If human subjects or materials from living humans are involved, completion of the requested information is essential to avoid delays in processing and reviewing the application. The Institutional Review Board (IRB) approval date must not be more than one year old.

The involvement of vertebrate animals requires that the necessary information be provided. The Institutional Animal Care and Use Committee (IACUC) approval of research protocols must not be more than three years old.

Total costs include indirect costs as well as direct costs.

Periods of support for domestic institutions should not exceed five years; for foreign applications, three years.

The bottom of the face page is to be signed by the responsible institutional official and the PI. "Per" signatures are not allowed. Not all federal scientists can apply for grant support. Therefore, an NIH scientist applying for support prior to leaving NIH to assume a position in a nonfederal institution must leave the Principal Investigator signature box blank and not sign the face-page at all.

Page 2: Description

Be realistic, clear, and concise. In as few words as possible, relate what you are going to do, how you are going to do it, and what you hope to accomplish. This most likely will be used verbatim or adapted for use as the Description section of the official agency record of the review committee's deliberations, the summary statement. Thus, avoid the use of personal pronouns and valuative or self-promoting statements.

Personnel

List *all* personnel, salaried or not, including consultants/collaborators and support staff, who will participate in the project. The information requested includes degrees, date of birth, and role in the project.

Page 3: Table of Contents

Completeness of this page is important for reviewers and staff to be able to find significant parts of the proposal quickly. This is especially the case in longer, more complex applications, such as the Program Project.

Page 4: Detailed Budget for Initial Budget Period

This section is one of the first that the reviewers will see in their reading of the application. Since this is the section that deals with the essential means to carry out the proposed project, it should be prepared with extreme care. A realistic, fully justified budget that indicates a knowledge of cost requirements, should be developed. Remember that the reviewers work in the same general area of science and know what it costs to do research. Obviously, grossly inflated budgets will raise questions about the PI's judgment.

Reviewers will note the total dollar support the PI is receiving for related or other projects. Therefore, to avoid arbitrary reductions, present the budget clearly and convincingly, with any hint of overlap with other funding fully explained. In over 85 percent of the applications, requested budgets are reduced by the reviewers.

Until 1987, when total costs (direct plus indirect) had to be inserted in items 7b and 8b on the face page, the reviewers only had a general awareness of indirect costs and little knowledge of an individual institution's indirect cost rates. Indirect costs are justified and legitimate charges that allow the institution to recoup its expenses in carrying out a government-sponsored project. The policy on indirect costs for colleges and universities has been established by OMB and is detailed in Circular A-21 (Office of Management and Budget, 1991). The policy for other nonprofit organizations is contained in Circular A-122 (1987).

The rates are negotiated between federal auditors and the institution administrators with no input from NIH. Reviewers are not supposed to consider indirect costs in arriving at their recommendations. The review staff will do its best to discourage any discussion of this matter and point out that reviewers must not penalize the PI for indirect cost rates over which they have no control. Indirect costs are not paid on foreign grants.

Items of importance are:

Direct costs only.

All personnel should be listed whether or not salaried. Each person's role in the project should be indicated; specific functions should be detailed on page 5 of the application under Justification.

In the third column (Type Appt.), list the number of months per year of the contractual appointment to the applicant organization. If an appointment is less than full time, indicate this with an asterisk and explain on page 5.

The percent effort to be expended on the project for each individual should be placed in the next column. This should be a realistic portion of the PI's total professional effort.

What percent will the PI expend? Too little effort will be suspect; 5 percent or less might indicate that person to be a proxy PI, which is unacceptable.

The fifth column (Inst. Base Salary) should contain the annual compensation paid for the individual's appointment. The applicant organization has the option of omitting this information; however,it may be requested by USPHS staff prior to award.

The salary requested (sixth column) cannot be greater than the base salary times the percent effort on the project. If a lesser amount is requested, this should be explained on page 5.

When the Veterans Administration (VA) is the applicant institution, salary support may not be requested for VA employees, and indirect costs are not permitted for federal agencies. The PI may indicate research effort on the projects up to 100 percent of the VA appointment. However, if the PI engages in nonresearch VA activities, this would reduce the level of effort on the proposed project.

VA employees with joint appointments at a university may apply for support in applications submitted by the university. The university's share of the investigator's salary may be requested. The activities at both organizations should comprise no more than 100 percent of the individual's professional activities.

In completing the detailed budget for the initial period, VA employees at a university should indicate the proportion of their university time in the Type Appt. column and the percent effort on the project and the institutional base salary compensated by the university in the appropriate columns. The salary requested cannot exceed the base salary times the percent effort. If effort from the VA activities also is to be devoted to the project, a separate line item for these columns should be completed to identify the individual's total effort to be applied to the project.

Currently, the amount of the direct salary awarded an individual cannot exceed $125,000 per year for 100 percent effort. This does not limit an individual's institutional salary, which may be supplemented with non-HHS funds. It is to be noted that the ceiling indicated above is set annually in accordance with the DHHS appropriation and is published in the *NIH Guide for Grants and Contracts*.

Applicant institutions may want to avail themselves of the option of not listing salaries and fringe benefits requested for some or all of the individuals listed on the budget page of the application. If they choose to omit these, asterisks should be substituted for the amounts in the original and six copies of the application. However, subtotals must still be inserted and a separate page 4 of the PHS 398 submitted with all salaries and benefits showing. This budget page will be used by internal staff only, who are instructed not to divulge the information to the reviewers.

Consultants should be named whether or not funds are sought for their participation. PIs should not list individuals they have not contacted. Include letters from consultants indicating their willingness to participate as well as the nature and extent of their consultation. If missing, it is quite likely that the review staff will request letters from the PI or may even contact the consultants directly.

If equipment requests are $500 or more, list the items to be purchased. The reviewers will know if a less expensive model of a particular piece of equipment is adequate. Therefore, avoid requesting funds for the premier model. Justification for these items should be provided on page 5.

If the supplies requested are less than $1,000, they do not have to be itemized, except for animals. Indicate the specific number and species of animals to be purchased.

Be realistic about travel requests and costs. Reviewers may recommend set amounts no matter where the PI is located. Indicate the number of trips, the purpose, and the individuals involved. Funds for foreign travel should be combined with the amounts for domestic travel. This request should be justified on page 5, describing the importance of travel to the objectives of the project.

Provide details regarding patient care costs also on page 5.

Itemize funds only for the alteration of existing facilities; new construction is not permissible.

The Other Expenses category can be used to list publication costs, computer charges, fee for service contracts, etc.

If the proposal is a consortium application involving a collaborating institution or contractual funds, it should include a separate budget for each participating organization. Indirect costs can be requested. Photocopies of unused pages 4 and 5 should be used to itemize the collaborating institutions' budgets. Note that both direct and indirect costs should be entered *after* the subtotal of direct costs for the initial budget period in these separate budgets. Pages should be numbered sequentially and inserted after pages 4 and 5.

Page 5: Budget for Entire Proposed Project Period

Space is provided on the bottom half of page 5 for the important and necessary justification of items that have been requested for all years, especially personnel and equipment. For example, if you have been doing ultrastructural cell research and request funds for a very expensive instrument, explain why the instrument you have been using will no longer be available and why a new or additional one is needed. There is a good chance you will not be unsuccessful in asking for a unique or expensive piece of equipment as long as you can make a sufficiently strong case for it. If the application is a competing renewal, justify any significant increases over current funding levels.

If you are requesting a major increase in effort and salary or adding personnel and equipment in future years, be sure to highlight this in the justification statement. This will avoid deletion of the items if reviewers seek to limit costs.

For Program Project (P01) applications, each subproject and core should have its own twelve-month and entire-period budgets in addition to the overall budget. Photocopies of unused pages 4 and 5 should be used for this purpose.

Page 6: Biographical Sketch

The important way to establish the qualifications and competence of the PI and the investigative group is in the content of the biographical sketches. This section should:

Contain sketches for all professional personnel, including consultants and collaborators, and be limited to two pages per individual.

Account for gaps or periods of inactivity or plans for a leave of absence during the proposed grant period. If you plan to be away from your home base for an extended period, make sure the scientific review administrator (SRA) is able to reach you or a knowledgeable associate while the proposal is under review.

List all publications during the past three years and any prior publications related to the research. These must include titles and the names of *all* the authors. To avoid exceeding the page limitations, list only the most relevant papers.

Page 7: Other Support

This page contains a comprehensive set of instructions and listing of items to be completed. Nothing should be left out. NIH has computer files of a PI's past USPHS grant, contract, and review experiences. These records are attached to the application when it is forwarded to the review committee office. In addition, NIH staff members maintain close contacts with their counterparts in other granting agencies, both government and private.

The list of other support must include proposals currently active, pending review, or pending funding and must be completed for all key professional personnel listed in the application. Include support from nonfederal sources, gifts, prizes, and other means available in direct support of research endeavors. If you are funded for similar work or have a related proposal pending funding or review, be sure to describe the differences, so that there can be no doubt about the possibility of overlapping support or duplicate funding.

It is important for you to protect yourself by being precise and clear about dates, dollar amounts, percent effort, and project aims for all support listed. This will avoid any reviewer misconceptions about the nature and extent of total support. Your signature and that of the appropriate institutional official at the bottom of the face page are supposed to guarantee that the information provided is accurate and complete.

However, it is wise to submit the same application to more than one granting organization, government or private. Especially in times of uncertain funding, one should cover "all bets." However, duplicate government funding for the same project is prohibited, and the Directorate of Biological Sciences of NSF will not accept applications also sent to NIH or the United States Department of Agriculture.

PIs should be aware, however, that simultaneous submissions of identical applications to different agencies within the USPHS, or to different institutes within an agency, will not be allowed. Important exceptions are an individual submitting a Research Career Development Award application who may propose the same research in a regular grant application and an individual who may submit a regular grant application essentially identical to a subproject that is part of a Program Project or Center grant application.

To avoid confusion caused by a profusion of detail and pages listing other support, it is suggested that a summary table similar to the accompanying chart be added to this part of the application:

Other Support

Grant Number	PI	Effort (%)	Current Year Award	Project Dates
Current				
1. CA54321-03[a]	Smith	30	$200,000	9/1/87–8/31/92
2. AI23456-05[b]	Smith	30	$180,000	2/1/87–1/31/92
3. AI20000-02	Jones	5	$150,000	7/1/89–6/30/92
4. Ill. Cancer Society[c]	Smith	10	$10,000	1/1/90–12/31/92
Pending Review				
5. CA55555-01[d]	Smith	35	$500,000[e]	12/1/90–11/30/93

[a]The present application is a renewal of this grant.

[b]This grant will terminate before the review of the present application. No renewal is contemplated.

[c]This grant cannot be renewed.

[d]Also submitted to NSF

[e]Total direct costs requested.

Page 8: Resources and Environment

Describe in detail the facilities that would be available specifically to the PI for the proposed project. Completeness is essential here, especially in describing supporting departments and clinical and animal facilities. It is important to indicate the proximity of the facilities to the main site of the research and the extent of their availability to the investigators. The lack of permanent space and equipment could signal a lack of support and commitment for the PI on the part of the institution and thus weaken the proposal. If facilities in other organizations or institutions are to be used, attach letters of commitment to the application.

Checklist

In completing the Checklist, be realistic in stating whether the proposal is new, a competing continuation, or a revision of a previously submitted application. Obviously a first-time application is new, while an application that includes new scientific directions and methodology for a project that is being funded usually is not a new application but a competing continuation application. A rewrite, even one with modified aims, of a recently submitted but unfunded application (usually within one year) is a revision. You must also indicate if the application is a supplemental proposal (request for additional funds to supplement a funded grant), represents a change in PI of a funded grant, or is a foreign application. If unsure, check with the Referral Section of DRG or ICD program staff. The Checklist also contains a number of assurances and certifications that are required as appropriate. These relate to:

Human Subjects	Delinquent Federal Debt
Vertebrate Animals	Misconduct in Science
Inventions and Patents	Civil Rights
Debarment and Suspension	Handicapped Individuals
Drug-Free Workplace (new or revised	Sex Discrimination
new applications only)	Age Discrimination
Lobbying	Program Income

The Checklist will not be duplicated with the rest of the application and will be used by PHS staff only. The Checklist must be the last page of the application and should be numbered accordingly.

Personal Data

Completion of this page is optional. There is a checkoff box for those who do not want to provide some or all of the information. If submitted, it should not be duplicated by the applicant, but attached to the signed original of the application after the Checklist. It will not be duplicated with the rest of the application at NIH and will not be part of the review process. Its purpose is to aid the PHS in monitoring the review and award process and to provide information about the nature and makeup of scientists who apply for federal funding.

Introduction

All amended and supplemental applications must have an Introduction (no more than three pages for the amended and one page for the supplemental).

Amended (Revised) Applications

If the application is a revision, you should indicate in the Introduction how the application has been changed to reflect agreement or disagreement with the prior review and any new data accumulated since the last submission. Reviewers appreciate a scholarly, documented account of the PI's point of view. Do not include undue negativism, sarcasm, and unnecessary argumentation, since these usually are not well received and could adversely affect the outcome of the review.

Examples abound of thoughtlessly revised proposals. One recent example involved an amended application that had been previously disapproved. The PI filled the Introduction Section with angry remarks directed at a member of the study section with whom he had previous scientific differences. He was contacted before the meeting by staff and informed that this was inappropriate and quite likely disadvantageous. Besides, that particular study section member was on sabbatical and not present at the review meeting in question. The long, painful silence was broken by an embarrassed, "What should I do?" He was advised to submit replacement pages with a more rational and better documented response to the previous Critique.

The revised text should be highlighted with bracketing, italics, indenting, or change in typography. Avoid submitting practically the same proposal, since an application marked "revised," but with no apparent revisions, or one that does not answer previous criticisms will be returned by NIH without further processing. In addition, it is unwise to quickly revise an application based on a verbal report of the review of the original proposal before you have seen the summary statement. It is unlikely that NIH will accept such an application.

Supplemental Applications

A supplemental award is meant only for a currently funded grant. Because of the length of time involved in the application process, it is likely that new information may be accumulated by the PI of a just-reviewed application, which would indicate that new or additional directions and methodologies should be pursued. This might tempt you to submit a supplemental application requesting additional funds even before a funding decision has been made on the original proposal. Such an application will not be accepted until an award has been made. For a currently funded grant, explain how the supplement, or lack of it, will affect the aims, experimental design, and methodology of the project. Competitive supplemental requests are not appropriate if the purpose is to restore funds that were reduced administratively or by downward negotiation. If the request is to restore funds deleted by the review panel, the PI must respond to the criticisms of the reviewers, and revisions in the application must be evident and clearly stated.

Research Plan

Up to this point, the application will contain mostly administrative information. The creative portion, the heart of the proposal, will be the Research Plan. Items 1–4

(Specific Aims through Experimental Design and Methods) are limited to a total of twenty-five pages, allocated at the PI's discretion, but must include all tables and graphs.

1. Specific Aims

These should be focused and clear. What are the long-term objectives of the research and what is to be accomplished? One page is recommended.

2. Background and Significance

What is the background of the present proposal? Evaluate existing knowledge, identifying gaps that will be filled by the project. A good understanding of the literature is expected, but the literature review need not be exhaustive. Describe the importance of the research and present a valid and testable hypothesis. This point is one the reviewers look for. Relate this section to the Aims and be careful not to exceed two to three pages.

3. Progress Report/Preliminary Studies

A progress report is required for competing continuation and supplemental applications. The reviewers will want to know if the earlier confidence in the PI was warranted by noting the extent of progress made toward achieving objectives. Summarize those aims and provide an account of published and unpublished results, indicating their importance. Publications and manuscripts submitted or accepted for publication should be listed, but reprints do not substitute for this report. Note that this list is excluded from the twenty-five-page limit. However, these materials (not more than ten items) may be submitted as part of the Appendix. The fate of a competing continuation application usually depends as much on past accomplishments as on future plans.

For new applications, provide appropriate preliminary data and experimental results as well as any other information that indicates that the hypothesis is reasonable and testable and that establishes your ability to pursue the proposed research. Include no more than ten reprints in the Appendix. (Five sets of the Appendix are required.) Six to eight pages are recommended for the narrative portion of Section 3.

4. Research Design and Methods

A well-defined problem deserves a well-defined approach. Provide details on the experimental design, methodology, and the means by which data will be collected and analyzed. It is here that details on human research protocols are presented, including a description of the composition of the proposed study population in terms of gender and racial/ethnic groups and the rationale for its choice. Also provide animal experimentation protocols. Describe any new methodology to be used and its advantages.

If there are multiple approaches to a problem, e.g., a number of different statistical instruments that can be used in a particular behavioral study, explain the rationale for your choice. It is important to discuss any potential problems, pitfalls, or limitations and the means to overcome them. The reviewers will be aware of the difficulties of a particular type of research and will want to know your understanding and awareness. Tables, figures, or copies of glossy photographs should be included. They should be well designed, with clear titles and footnotes to enhance the point being made.

Reviewers have been criticized for not recognizing or appreciating "innovative" research. However, it is your responsibility to show in this section that the ideas and approaches are indeed innovative and offer advantages over existing approaches and methodologies. Take the opportunity here to present your case for innovation and uniqueness, not after the review has taken place.

There are no specific page limitations for this section, but remember that sections 1–4 must not exceed 25 pages.

5. Human Subjects

Human subjects are involved when research materials or data are obtained from living, identifiable humans. This is not the case with the use of pooled blood samples, for example, which obviously could not be identified with specific individuals. While autopsy materials do not fall under federal regulations, applicants should be aware that the use of these materials is governed by state and local laws. The application should be completed in time for the research protocols involving human subjects to be reviewed by the IRB before being submitted to the NIH.

To satisfy PHS requirements and the review needs of the study section, you must address six points. If these are omitted or incomplete, the review of the application will be deferred. The PI must:

1. Provide details of the involvement of human subjects and characteristics of the subject population. Summarize the gender and racial/ethnic composition of the population and its health status. Identify the criteria for inclusion or exclusion of any subpopulation. If gender representation or inclusion of minorities is not addressed, provide a clear rationale for their exclusion. If special classes of subjects are to be involved, e.g., fetuses, pregnant women, prisoners, explain the rationale.
2. Identify the sources of research material to be obtained from living, identifiable humans in the form of specimens, records, or data.
3. Describe the plans for the recruitment of subjects and the consent procedures to be followed. Include the circumstances under which consent will be sought and obtained. The consent form, which must have IRB approval, should be submitted to the PHS *only* upon request. PI's should be forewarned that if the consent form is included in the original application package, it becomes "fair game" for evaluation by the reviewers.

4. Describe any potential risks, physical, psychological, social, legal, or other and assess their likelihood and seriousness. Describe any alternative procedures.
5. Describe the procedures for protecting against or minimizing any potential risks of harm. When appropriate, discuss provisions for ensuring necessary medical intervention in the event of adverse effects. Describe provisions to monitor data collected to ensure the safety of subjects.
6. Why are the risks reasonable in relation to anticipated benefits?

As detailed above and in Chapter 13, "Areas of Special Interest," all applications involving human subjects must give appropriate attention to the inclusion of women and minorities in study populations. For program project applications, the program director must address these issues for each subproject where human studies are involved. Review staff will seek such information, if missing. Review panel members will evaluate the attention paid to these matters. For foreign applications, this policy applies fully. However, since the definition of a minority differs in other countries, the applicant must discuss the relevance of research involving foreign population groups to the United States' populations, including minorities.

6. Vertebrate Animals

The humane care and use of laboratory animals in research are of prime importance. Procedures that do not conform to PHS policy and acceptable practices will lead to nonconsideration (disapproval) of the application. Principles that should be adhered to can be summarized as two broad rules:

The project should be worthwhile and justified on the basis of anticipated results for the good of society and the contribution to knowledge, and the work should be planned and performed by qualified scientists.

Animals should be confined, restrained, transported, cared for, and used in experimental procedures in a manner to avoid any unnecessary discomfort, pain, or injury. Special attention must be provided when the proposed research involves dogs, cats, nonhuman primates, large numbers of animals, or animals that are in short supply or are costly.

Here too, the application should be completed in time for the IACUC to review the research protocols involving vertebrate animals and still meet the appropriate receipt date for the application.

When animals are to be used, five points must be addressed in the application for the IACUC's review and the review by the study section (omission or incompleteness could lead to deferral). The PI must:

1. Provide a detailed description of the use of the animals. Identify the species, strains, ages, sex, and numbers to be used.
2. Justify the use, choice of species, and the number to be used. If the animals

are in short supply, costly, or to be used in large numbers, provide a rationale for their selection and quantity.

3. Describe the veterinary care to be provided.
4. Describe procedures to minimize discomfort, distress, pain, and injury. Describe the use of analgesic, anesthetic, and tranquilizing drugs or restraining devices.
5. Describe any method of euthanasia and the reasons for its selection. Is this method consistent with the recommendations of the American Veterinary Medical Association? If not, provide justification for not following recommendations.

Further details regarding the use of human subjects and vertebrate animals are discussed in Chapter 13.

7. Consultants/Collaborators

The right choice of consultants or collaborators will strengthen a proposal substantially, especially one from a first-time, relatively inexperienced investigator. However, in selecting consultants or collaborators, be aware that some are potential reviewers and their participation in the project would eliminate them from consideration. Letters from consultants/collaborators confirming their roles on the project should be attached to the application, not placed in the Appendix.

8. Consortium/Contractual Arrangements

If there is to be a major collaboration involved, it may be advantageous to submit the application with a consortium agreement. In this situation, in addition to the applicant, substantive programmatic work will be carried out by one or more cooperating institutions that are separate, legal entities independent of the applicant. Another option is to subcontract a portion of the research. Describe the nature of the agreements and attach letters signed by the proper officials of the collaborating organization(s). These statements should indicate that the collaborating institution(s) will follow the appropriate federal regulations and policies. If the collaborating organization's activities represent a major effort and portion of the project, explain why the applicant organization (and not the collaborating group) should be designated the grantee. In addition, the applicant organization may not serve as a conduit for an award to another party, especially if that party is ineligible to receive an award on its own.

9. Literature Cited

This is limited to six pages. It is important to show that you are aware of, and familiar with, the pertinent literature. Do not scatter references throughout the text, but list them here, in the last section of the Research Plan. Each literature citation must include the title, names of *all* authors, and the appropriate book or journal reference. The list may include, but may not replace, the list of publications in the Progress Report required for competing continuation and supplemental applications.

Appendix

The Appendix will not be duplicated with the rest of the application. Therefore, its distribution will be limited to the assigned NIH institute, the SRA's office file, and the assigned reviewers. A copy of the Appendix material will be made available to other members of the review panel whose expertise may be similar. Do not use the Appendix to avoid the page limitations of the application. If glossy photographs or other materials are submitted that cannot be copied in the body of the application, five collated sets should be included in the Appendix. Should the PI want any of this material saved and returned, this should be made known to the review staff. For competing continuation and supplemental applications, include no more than ten papers published, accepted, or submitted for publication related to, or resulting from, this project.

Review Criteria

In their reviews of R01 applications, the members of a study section will be looking for the following points, which should be kept fully in mind when preparing applications:

Significance and originality from a scientific and technical standpoint. Is it good science? Is it unique, novel, innovative? Are you investigating a subject that may be overly studied already?

Is the research descriptive of a phenomenon or does it attempt to explain the underlying mechanisms of the phenomenon under study? The latter proposals usually are more favorably received.

Adequacy of the methodology to carry out the research. Is the experimental approach appropriate? Have you shown you are capable of setting priorities? Are you aware of the obstacles and pitfalls and the alternatives to overcome them?

Qualifications and experience of the PI and staff. Have you adequately provided evidence of your knowledge of the field and competence to conduct the research? Is the proposal current with regard to the literature in the field? Have you indicated an ability to be self critical?

Reasonable availability of resources.

Reasonableness of the proposed budget and project period.

Protection of human subjects, animals, and the environment. Careful consideration of the inclusion of women and minorities in the study population; and the lack of biohazardous procedures.

Preliminary data or satisfactory progress and a testable hypothesis are essential ingredients of successful applications.

FIRST INDEPENDENT RESEARCH SUPPORT AND TRANSITION (FIRST) AWARD

This award is meant to provide a sufficient period of support (five years) for newly independent investigators at domestic institutions to initiate their own research and demonstrate the merit of their research ideas. The eligibility criteria are:

The PI must be independent of a mentor, yet at the beginning stages of a research career.

No more than five years must have elapsed since the completion of postdoctoral research training. Those in the final stages of training may apply, but no award will be made to those in training.

You must otherwise be eligible at the applicant institution to serve as a PI on a traditional research project grant (R01).

You must not have been a PI on any PHS-supported project other than a Small Grant (R03), AREA Grant (R15), or Research Career Awards (K series) directed principally to physicians, dentists, or veterinarians. Current or past Research Career Development Awardees (K04) are not eligible. PIs of subprojects on Program Project Grants (P01), Center Grants, or Minority Biomedical Research Support Grants (S06) may be eligible. These individuals should contact the extramural activities staff of the relevant ICD for further information.

Five years of support must be requested and the PI must commit no less than 50 percent effort to the proposed project. Up to 100 percent may be requested, however.

A letter from a department head or dean must be included in the application addressing the eligibility and suitability of the proposed PI to lead a research project and whether the individual would be qualified to be a PI on an R01 grant.

Three letters of reference are required. Request these well in advance of the application receipt date so they can be attached to the front of the application in envelopes *sealed by the referee*. NIH is likely to return an application without the three letters.

Since the award is meant for persons with minimal experience, applicants with well-demonstrated experience and competence should be aware that they might be considered overqualified. Thus, you should be very clear about your research status and your need for this award at the current stage of your career. The grant is not renewable. However, the research can be continued and extended by applying for an R01 grant award.

MODIFICATIONS FOR THE RESEARCH CAREER
DEVELOPMENT AWARD (RCDA) APPLICATION

The PHS 398 is used also for the RCDA application. This prestigious award, by providing full or partial salary support, is intended to foster the development of scientists who have demonstrated outstanding potential for independent research careers. It is not intended for senior investigators who have attained associate or full professorial rank and have published extensively. Consultation with the appropriate staff of the awarding components before writing or submitting an application is encouraged to clarify any matters relating to eligibility, review, or award. Additional instructions are provided in the application kit and should be followed to avoid delays. Several points should be noted, however.

The candidate must be a U.S. citizen, noncitizen national, or lawfully admitted permanent resident.

The candidate should normally have at least five years of postdoctoral research experience, including two years as the PI of a peer-reviewed research grant. Those not meeting the experience criterion must provide evidence, in the application, that they have achieved an equivalent level of experience and independence to qualify.

At least 80 percent of the individual's time must be committed to research. Also, the sponsoring institution must include in the application a guarantee that, if an award is made, the candidate will have full time available for research and research-related activities (research training, clinical activities, teaching related to research goals, etc.).

The candidate should summarize both short-term and long-term career plans and indicate how the award will enhance research development.

For an award to be made, the candidate must show at the time of the award that there is independent funding sufficient for the research proposed in the application. The support may be from institutional or outside sources.

The RCDA is not a device to acquire departmental salaries. The applicant organization must describe fully its plans for the candidate's future support and career development, including status in the department, plans for supervision, and guidance and opportunities for training and interaction with other researchers.

A letter should be submitted by the candidate's department chair describing plans for the candidate at the conclusion of the RCDA period and indicating how the candidate would spend the next five years should an award be made, versus how the time would be spent in the case of no award. Emphasis in this letter should be placed on how an award would contribute to the candidate's research career.

For candidates already in full-time research, especially strong and convincing justification is required to show that the award would indeed enhance career development.

No more than six publications and manuscripts submitted or accepted for publication may be submitted with new applications.

Review Criteria

In reviewing an RCDA application, the study section members will evaluate the following areas:

- The quality and extent of the candidate's education, scientific training, and research experience
- The candidate's research career potential as a creative, independent investigator
- The merit of the proposed research including its significance and originality
- The adequacy of the research environment in terms of the availability of space and equipment resources, facilities, technical assistance, and opportunities for critical professional interaction with senior colleagues
- The ability of the plan to enhance the candidate's career development. Is there an institutional commitment that will permit the candidate to spend essentially full time in the actual conduct of research and research-related activities?

OTHER MODIFICATIONS

The PHS 398 is used also to apply for the Program Project grant (P01) and for the Institutional National Research Service Award (T32). Specific instructions are provided to complete these applications either in the PHS 398 kit, a particular Request for Applications (RFA), or from NIH institutes that publish their own instructions for the P01. Applicants are advised to communicate with appropriate ICD staff before completing and submitting any application for a solicited or unsolicited program project grant.

REQUESTS FOR APPLICATIONS (RFA)

Applications submitted in response to RFAs should have the specific label (look for it in the application kit) attached to the face page for quick identification and rapid processing. Every RFA will have special instructions for submitting proposals, and these should be followed closely.

In almost all cases, there is a single receipt date specified. Applications not meeting that deadline either will be returned or will be allowed to compete with the general run of applications received at the next receipt date. Whether the latter option applies is stated in the RFA and usually depends on the type of application requested. In most cases, review is done by a Special Emphasis Panel (SEP).

PHS 416–1

This PHS application form is used to apply for an NRSA Individual Postdoctoral Fellowship (F32) or Senior Fellowship (F33).

INDIVIDUAL POSTDOCTORAL FELLOWSHIP AWARD

The application should be developed in collaboration with the sponsor. However, it is essential that it reflect the thoughts and ideas of the applicant, not of the sponsor. To shorten the period applicants have to wait for decisions on funding, the applications are reviewed in an expedited manner (approximately four months from receipt to possible award). The receipt dates are January 10, May 10, and September 10. Complete applications are mandatory to avoid delays.

Review panels meet in March, July, and November. Second level review is by ICD staff fellowship committees, which meet in May, September, and January. Council review is not required. Thus, the time from receipt date to funding decision is approximately 20 weeks. Previously the period was approximately 44 weeks as in the current case of a usual R01 application. DRG publishes a separate "Helpful Hints" for fellowship applicants (Division of Research Grants, National Institutes of Health, 1990. *Helpful Hints on Preparing a Fellowship Application to the National Institutes of Health*. Bethesda, MD.). As in the case of the PHS 398, computer-generated facsimiles may be substituted for the government-printed form. No deviations from that form are acceptable. Also, type size limitations must be followed. Be sure to follow the directions in the application kit.

REVIEW CRITERIA

The criteria focus on four main components of the application:

- *Applicant:* Education, honors, experience, publications, references, and training and career goals
- *Research proposal:* Originality, scientific merit, and training potential
- *Training resources and environment:* Will the training situation provide the best conditions and opportunities for the training?
- *Sponsor:* Is the training project in the sponsor's area of expertise and does the sponsor have the time for adequate supervision of the applicant? Has the sponsor successfully trained other research scientists?

THE APPLICATION

Part I is to be filled out by the applicant while the sponsor completes Part II. Both parts must be submitted in the same envelope.

References

Individuals asked to submit references must be listed with their institutional affiliations on page 3 (Table of Contents). The reference reports are the responsibility of the applicant. The NIH review staff may or may not send reminders that these have not been submitted. At least three must accompany the application in envelopes *sealed by the referees* and attached to the face page of the original copy of the application. The lack of sufficient references could result in deferral of the processing and review, or withdrawal of the application. If the application is a revised version or a competing continuation, new reference forms must be submitted.

Referees should be chosen carefully. Select only those individuals who can provide meaningful evaluations and who are certain to return the completed forms to you in time to meet the proper receipt date. If the thesis advisor or chief of service is not submitting a reference report, a reason should be given. It is possible that the review staff will seek information on this point. Do not use the sponsor of the current fellowship application as a reference. Avoid delay by requesting referees to use black ink for their reference reports. Blue does not reproduce well in many copiers.

Part I: Face Page

Level of Fellowship

Note that the Senior Fellowship (F33) applicant must have possessed a doctoral degree for at least seven years and have already established a research career. This senior award is meant for individuals wishing to make a major career change or to acquire new research capabilities and is not designed for persons seeking to prove their research potential. Also, no individual, whether seeking postdoctoral research training support or a more senior award, may receive more than a total of three years of any type of NRSA support.

Citizenship

Applicants must be citizens of the United States, noncitizen nationals, or permanent residents at the time of application. It is necessary for a noncitizen to submit with the application a notarized statement that the applicant possesses an Alien Registration Receipt Card (I-151 or I-551).

Page 2

Education, Employment, Sponsor, Research Proposal Description

List all employment after completion of college. Be sure to account for all time, including periods of unemployment. This information is important for determining the stipend amount. For all postdoctoral individuals receiving support through institutional or individual NRSAs, the annual stipends are based on years of relevant experience. They range from $18,600 (0 years) to $32,300 (7 or more years). Senior Fellowship applicants need only list employment following completion of the doctoral degree.

In relating the proposed research training to career goals, be realistic, indicating where you expect to pursue your career (government, academia, industry, etc.). Senior fellows should list education as appropriate and omit information on the thesis.

In the description of the proposed research, be concise about the objectives and aims of the research, indicating its health relatedness as well as its training potential. This section may be used as the Description in the summary statement.

Page 4

Scholastic Performance

Types of courses taken and grades received are indications of the training and competence of the applicant and are part of the review process. This section should be omitted by Senior Fellowship applicants.

Page 5

Honors, Thesis Advisor/Chief of Service, Concurrent Support

List concurrent support applied for or planned during this same period. If there is related support from other sources, explain and indicate the need for further funding. Also, it would be helpful to indicate your work priorities if support is being applied for or exists for other projects.

Page 6

Research Experience, Revised Application, Research Training Plans

List all publications and include manuscripts submitted or in preparation. List *all* authors. Submit three sets of the most significant publications. Competing continuation applications should include three sets of all publications resulting from the current NRSA support. If the application is revised, specify significant changes and present a properly reasoned rebuttal to the Critique of the previous review, if you disagree with it. Be scholarly and not argumentative. Present new data, if available. Be aware that if no revisions are apparent, the application is likely to be returned.

For candidates with the Ph.D. degree, the research training plan probably is the most essential part of the application. All of the academic courses and previous training mean little if the proposed research has little scientific merit and is thus of little training potential. Candidates with the M.D. degree only, however, may not have had much research experience and generally are not expected to present as sophisticated a research plan as those with the Ph.D. This will be taken into account in the review of the application.

In developing the research training plan with the sponsor, indicate what will be done each year of the fellowship, specifying percentages of time for each activity (research, course work, etc.). Discuss the training potential and significance of the research. The sections on Specific Aims, Background and Significance, Research Design and Methods, and Literature Citations together are limited to ten pages. The explanations, procedures, rules, and regulations regarding human subjects and vertebrate animals, which were presented earlier in this chapter and appear later in Chapter 13, must be followed.

Indicate the respective contributions of the sponsor and of the applicant in the preparation of the application, *not* in accomplishing the research. Explain the choice of sponsor and institution, especially in terms of the research training opportunities available. If the plans are to remain at the doctoral or current institution or with the same mentor, explain why further training at that site or with that person would be desirable. This is also true for applicants for Senior Fellowships. If the request is to train at a foreign institution, explain what special opportunities are offered that are not available in the United States.

Personal Data Page

As in the case of the PHS 398, this page is optional and, if submitted, should not be duplicated by the applicant but attached to the signed original copy of the application after the Checklist.

Checklist

Applicants should complete section I-A and B. In addition, Senior Fellowship applications should include completed section I-C. The sponsor will complete section II. As with the PHS 398, there are a number of assurances/certifications that must be provided. The Checklist will not be duplicated with the rest of the application.

Part II: Face Page

Items 9–14 should be completed by the sponsor. These include information on human subjects, vertebrate animals, and the institution(s) involved in the training. The same rules apply for these items as outlined for applicants for research grants.

Pages 7 and 8

Biographical Sketch of Sponsor

This is limited to two pages. If the sponsor has recently completed a biographical sketch for a PHS 398, these pages may be substituted. In the case of a co-sponsor or advisor, include that person's sketch as well.

Sponsor's Research and Training Support

As in the case of the PHS 398, list and describe all active and pending support to include gifts and prizes. Identify the research support funds that will be available to the applicant during the period of the proposed fellowship award.

Sponsor's Previous Fellows/Trainees

The sponsor should provide the total number of pre- and postdoctoral individuals and provide information on a representative five. This should include their present organizations and titles or occupations.

Page 9

Facilities and Commitment

The quality of the environment under which the research training will take place is a very significant factor in the review of the application. The training environment and available research facilities and equipment should be described. The reviewers will want to know what plans the sponsor has for the fellow during the tenure of the fellowship. If human subjects or vertebrate animals will be involved in the research, the six points for human subjects, including information regarding gender/minority representation, and the five points for animals (detailed earlier) must be completed. Without this information or proper certification and approval, the review of the application may be deferred. There may not be any reminders from review staff.

Service Requirement

Award recipients must agree to engage in biomedical or behavioral health-related research or health-related teaching within two years after termination of the fellowship for a continuous period equal to the total NRSA support in excess of 12 months. For example, a Fellow with 24 months of support, would have to serve for 12 months.

Payback Provision

If fellows fail to comply with the service agreement, they must return money to the federal government. The amount is set by a formula that takes into account the total amount of financial support received, the amount awarded in the first 12 months, the total number of months of obligation, and the number of months served in payback effort.

PHS 6246–1

Phase I-SBIR Award (R43)

The Omnibus Solicitation publication of the PHS contains the application form and instructions for the SBIR. A copy can be obtained by calling the Office of Grants Inquiries of DRG at (301)496–7441 (also see Chapter 14). In general, the same rules and procedures apply to the preparation of an application for a Phase I SBIR award as to the completion of the PHS 398 for a research project grant. However, there is a twenty-five-page limit for the *entire* SBIR application; no Appendix is permitted. The receipt dates are April 15, August 15, and December 15.

Face Page

Principal Investigator

The eligibility for this award rests heavily on the status of the PI. More than one-half of the PI's time must be spent with the applicant organization at the time of the award and during the conduct of the project. Documentation must be submitted with the application to verify the PI's eligibility. Upon receipt of applications, an NIH committee is convened to judge eligibility; usually a small, but significant, number of applicants are asked to furnish further proof. Most problems are created when an academic person sets up or works with a commercial venture. This relationship and commitment must be made clear.

Human Subjects/Vertebrate Animals

In the case of research involving human subjects and vertebrate animals, most applicant organizations will not have an IRB or IACUC, and some may not even have proper facilities for such research. Therefore, they must show that they or collaborating organizations will comply with all pertinent regulations. Form 596, "Protection of Human Subjects, Assurance/Certification/Declaration," is included for this purpose in the Solicitation. By filing an Animal Welfare Assurance with the NIH, the applicant organization commits itself to follow the rules, regulations, and practices stipulated in the PHS policy.

Work Site

If more than one work site is involved, one must be the applicant organization.

Small Business Certification

Be sure to complete this section being aware of the definition of a small business:

- Organized for profit, independently owned, not dominant in its field, principal place of business in the United States
- At least 51 percent owned by U.S. citizen or permanent resident alien
- Number of employees does not exceed 500

Proprietary Information

The inclusion of proprietary information in an SBIR application always poses a problem. Applicants should avoid including such information *unless* it is absolutely necessary for proper evaluation of the proposal. While the review staff will stress the confidentiality of the review process, and the PHS will do everything possible to protect such information, applicants should be aware of the limitations of protection when the application must be reviewed by staff and experts serving on review committees and advisory councils. Most of the reviewers work in the fields represented by the proposals and some might come from the small business community.

Page 2

Abstract of Research Plan

As required by the R01 application, relate what you aim to do, how you are going to do it, and what you hope to accomplish. Be concise and specific. The Abstract most likely will be used as the Description for the summary statement.

Page 3

Budget

Direct plus indirect costs normally may not exceed $50,000 for a period normally no longer than six months. Only under special circumstances, negotiated with program staff of the funding ICD, can this period be extended for a limited time. Also, consultant and contractual costs may not exceed 33 percent of the total costs.

REVIEW CRITERIA

In reviewing applications, the members of the study section will evaluate:

- The soundness and technical merit of the proposed research
- The potential of the research for technological innovation
- The qualifications of the PI, supporting staff, and consultants
- The adequacy and suitability of the facilities and research environment
- The appropriateness of the requested budget
- The adequacy of the protection of human subjects, animals, and the environment

PHS 6246–2

PHASE II: SBIR AWARD (R44)

The objective of this award is to continue the research or research and development efforts initiated in a Phase I award. The application may not be submitted prior to the end of the Phase I budget period. Application forms are sent to phase I grantees by the Referral Office of DRG.

The receipt dates are the same as for Phase I: April 15, August 15, and December 15. The application must be submitted within the first three receipt dates following the expiration of the Phase I budget period. If the application is a revised or amended version of an earlier submission, it must be submitted on the first receipt date following the official notification that the original application is not to be funded. Finally, no award for a Phase II grant can be made until the Status Report for Phase I has been received. There can be only one Phase II award per SBIR project.

Eligibility

Since an award can only be made to a Phase I grantee, eligibility requirements are the same. The work must be performed in its entirety in the United States and cannot be for market research.

REVIEW CRITERIA

The reviewers will evaluate:

- The degree to which Phase I objectives were met and feasibility demonstrated
- The potential of the proposed research for technological innovation

- The technical, economic, or societal importance of the problem or opportunity and anticipated benefits, if successful
- The adequacy of Phase II objectives and methodology for addressing the problem or opportunity
- The scientific and technical merit of the research, with special emphasis on its innovation or originality
- The qualifications of the PI, supporting staff, and consultants
- The reasonableness of the budget
- The adequacy and suitability of the facilities and the research environment
- The adequacy of the protection of human subjects, animals, and the environment

Much of the application form is similar to the PHS 398, and the same preparation principles should be utilized.

Face Page

Period of Requested Support

Normally the period of support may not exceed two years. Exceptions may be made following negotiation with staff of the funding ICD.

Costs

The total costs for the Phase II period should not exceed $500,000. Awards of larger amounts and for longer periods may be made in cases where the USPHS funding agency's mission needs or research plans justify such exceptions.

Page 4

Twelve Month Budget

Consultant and contractual costs may not exceed 50 percent of the total costs requested.

Research Plan

Sections A–E, Specific Aims through Experimental Design and Methods, are limited to thirty pages. These sections must contain a Phase I Final Report and a tentative timetable for the Phase II research.

Literature Cited

This section is limited to four pages.

Appendix

Three sets are requested.

PHS 2590

This application form is automatically sent to grantees just prior to yearly anniversary award dates. It is used to request noncompeting continuation support. Comprehensive completion of this form is the grantee's opportunity to let program staff know of progress, accomplishments, and future plans (see Chapter 11). It does not replace the PHS 398 for competing continuation applications and is not seen by reviewers during competing continuation reviews.

PHS 5161–1

Grants can be made by the agencies of the PHS to state and local governments. When applying for support, use PHS 5161–1 or, if desired, use PHS 398. Referral Office staff prefers the 398.

6

The Referral System

The policy of the NIH requires that grant applications, with few exceptions, be received centrally by DRG. The grant decision process begins in the Referral Office. This office's responsibility for the receipt, processing, and referral of grant applications extends beyond NIH in that other PHS organizations with grant programs, such as the ADAMHA utilize these services.

The NIH practice of controlling the initial flow of applications into the system has proved to be a wise policy because of the enormous growth and proliferation of the programs and grant mechanisms over the years, the imposition of new policies and procedures on the system, and the increased volume of applications. Some of the advantages accruing to the NIH for maintaining a central office responsible for receipt and referral of applications are:

1. Central receipt has permitted more efficient application processing, utilizing standard and consistent procedures. Applications can be easily located and rules, such as adherence to deadline dates, uniformly implemented.
2. Since the program interests of the various NIH awarding units are broad and in many cases overlapping, decisions are made by knowledgeable and neutral referees, protective of the interests of all NIH awarding units.
3. Central receipt assures capture of data from all submitted applications in a timely and orderly way. The NIH data system is used to generate reports for analytic purposes and lists required by review groups at almost every step in the grants process.

The volume of competing applications has increased substantially over the years. Table 6.1 indicates the magnitude of the competing application workload managed by the Referral Office.

The three-cycle-a-year review schedule has been followed almost from the beginning of the grant program in the late 1940s. The purpose is to obtain a more even distribution of the workload. However, the burden on the referral system has steadily grown due to the increased number of submissions, proliferation of RFAs, and development of new mechanisms of support, many of which have different receipt dates. Thus the Referral Office receives applications continuously. The

TABLE 6.1. Volume of Competing Applications

Fiscal Year	Reviewed by USPHS	Reviewed by NIH	Reviewed by DRG
1975	23,176	16,916	15,099
1980	26,396	21,105	18,661
1985	31,807	28,470	23,625
1986	29,955	26,885	22,486
1987	33,804	28,841	22,958
1988	32,771	28,888	23,089
1989	34,735	29,121	24,111
1990	36,714	29,529	24,314
1991 (estimate)	37,752	30,332	24,846

current receipt dates and key dates in the review cycles for the prominent application types are outlined in Tables 6.2 and 6.3, respectively.

The Referral Office is organized into two units, one responsible for processing applications and the other for assigning applications. The well-organized staff of these units manage the workload with amazing efficiency. The loss of even a single application in this huge mass of paper is a rare occurrence. To highlight the referral process, tracing the flow of a single application through the various steps should prove not only instructive but also serve as a means of offering suggestions in dealing with this key decision-making office.

INITIAL PROCESSING

Receipt Date

Applications are received in the DRG mail room and date-stamped. Instructions in the PHS 398 kit tell the sender to retain the mailing-date receipt from the postal service or express service. Deadline dates falling on a weekend or holiday are automatically extended to the next working day. Missing a deadline can be a serious matter, because it means a decision on the application will be delayed approximately four months. In the case of a late submission, there are opportunities available to avoid delays.

1. Request a waiver of deadline in a covering letter when the application is formally submitted, but not before. The letter must offer a reasonable explanation for the delay. Reasonable explanations are personal illness, family illness, staffing problems, or other realistic and convincing reasons.

TABLE 6.2. Application Receipt Dates for Unsolicited Grant Applications

January 10	February 1	March 1
May 10	June 1	July 1
September 10	October 1	November 1

	Research Grant applications	Research Grant applications
	New	Competing Continuation
		Supplemental
		Revised
	Program Project and Center Grant applications	
	New	
	Competing Continuation	
	Supplemental	
	Revised	
National Research Service Award applications	Research Career Development Award applications	
New	New	
Competing Continuation	Revised	
Supplemental		
Revised		

Unsolicited AIDs applications for expedited review	January 2 or May 1 or September 1
	For new, competing continuation, supplemental, and revised
Academic Research Enhancement Award (AREA) applications	June 22
RFAs	Receipt dates are specified in the RFA announcement

2. In addition to the above, if you have been working with the NIH program staff on an application, they may be willing to submit a memo to the Referral Office requesting favorable consideration of your waiver.

In any event, although the NIH policy is to adhere to the published receipt dates, in reality the staff is sympathetic and will make every reasonable attempt to accept a late application. Final waiver decisions reside with the DRG staff and are directly related to the workload and the length of the delay. Because funding decisions must occur no later than six months after receipt, applicants should not expect DRG to accept late AIDS applications.

TABLE 6.3. Key Dates in Each Review Cycle

Application Receipt Dates	Review Group Meetings	Advisory Council Meetings	Earliest Start Date
January 10* February 1 March 1	June/July	Sept./Oct.	Dec. 1
May 10* June 1 July 1	Oct./Nov.	Jan./Feb.	April 1
September 10* October 1 November 1	Feb./March	May/June	July 1
For individual fellowship applications			
January 10	Feb./March	N/A	June 1
May 10	June/July	N/A	October 1
September 10	Oct./Nov.	N/A	February 1
For unsolicited, investigator-initiated AIDS applications			
January 2	March	May/June	July 1
May 1	July	Sept./Oct.	November 1
September 1	November	Jan./Feb.	March 1

*Institutional National Research Service Award applications.

Name Check

From the mail room, the application proceeds to a records unit which captures data from the face page. This enables a name search to be conducted of the PI's records, using the NIH grant and contract data system. The system will retrieve:

Information related to each active grant, no matter what the type (e.g., R01, P01, F32, T32, K04, etc.). The most relevant items are the grant number, grant title, the name of the study section or institute review committee that conducted the scientific review, priority score/percentile, dates of project period, and dollar amounts recommended/awarded for each year.

Similar information for each pending application already in the system, but with an incomplete review outcome

Similar information for each approved but unfunded application

Similar information for each application disapproved within the last three grant cycles

Multiple submissions by the same PI for the same grant cycle

Information related to each cooperative agreement

Information related to each active contract

Membership on NIH committees. The file will identify the name of the committee and the date a member's appointment will terminate.

Principal investigators should be aware of the importance of accurately reporting all other support as instructed in the application form. A name search is not able to identify a PI's grant support if he is listed as a participant in a secondary role on an R01 or a subproject director on a P01 or center grant. However, there is a very good chance that an alert program or review staff member will be aware of such support.

REFERRAL DECISIONS

The application, along with grant and contract history records and any correspondence or internal memos received prior to its submission, is sent next to the Assignment Section of the Referral Office for action by the professional staff. The Referral Office is managed by a chief and three assistant chiefs. The Assignment Section consists of twelve referral officers who also are senior scientific review administrators (SRAs) of DRG study sections. In addition to the DRG staff, the Referral Office includes professional staff from other PHS components serviced by this office.

The applications are initially subjected to a "gross sort" by the assistant chiefs to remove applications intended for other agencies. NIH applications to be reviewed by ICD committees are identified and referral decisions made by the assistant chiefs. The remaining majority of the applications will be reviewed by DRG study sections. Based on an initial perusal, the assistant chiefs forward applications for more careful reading and referral decisions to the referral officers. Each referral officer is assigned approximately ten study sections, usually in closely related disciplines or specialty areas.

The decisions to be made are:

a. Health-relatedness

The scientific content and goals should be related to the mission of the NIH. This determination is not time consuming because of the small numbers of questionable applications and the liberal attitude of the agency. However, NIH applications intended to support services without a research component are usually returned.

b. Completeness

Incomplete applications are returned, as well as those not adhering to the page limitations or other instructions, such as format or type size.

c. Institute Assignment

An NIH sponsor for the application must be designated based on matching application content with the program interests of an institute. In cases of overlapping program interests, an application can be assigned to two institutes for funding consideration. If the interests of more than two institutes are significantly involved, the application is usually assigned to the NIGMS.

d. Study Section Assignment

The nature of the science dictates the assignment (see Appendix 4 for guidelines). In the case of competing continuations and supplements, the referral ordinarily is to the same study section that reviewed the original application. K04s and R01s from the same investigator are referred to the same study section. A study section is not permitted to review applications from one of its own members. Applications from study section members are either referred to another closely related study section or to a special study section. Amended (revised) applications are returned usually twice to the same study section that conducted the original review. If more than one year has elapsed from the time of the initial submission, the application normally will get a new grant number and a new study section assignment.

The PI's previous grant history may influence the referral. While the majority of applications find a study section home without too much difficulty, there are a significant number of problem cases which require discussion with other referral officers and SRAs before they can be properly assigned.

e. Application Type

Is the application new, a competing continuation, a supplement, an amended application, or a response to an RFA or a PA? Many times an application designated as new by the PI is really a competing continuation with a different title. The reasons for this are uncertain but may be due to a change in research direction, to investigators claiming every application is new, or to avoid complying with the requirements for a progress report. Such nuances may be difficult for the system to detect initially but may be identified later by an alert SRA or program staff member.

f. Amended (Revised) Applications

Amended applications submitted without significant change are usually returned, either at this point or after additional reading by the study section SRA. Amended applications submitted the cycle following the original review are carefully scrutinized to determine if they have been sufficiently modified to be accepted.

Reference sources used by referral officers in making decisions are:

Referral Guidelines for Funding Components of PHS: This document describes in considerable detail the program interests of all PHS funding components.

Referral Guidelines for Initial Review Groups of NIH: This document describes the scientific review capability of each DRG study section and institute review committee.

Grant history records obtained from the NIH data system

Conflict-of-interest policy in the case of applications from committee members

Correspondence from the investigator requesting assignment to a particular study section or institute

Memos from the NIH program staff requesting an institute assignment or perhaps pointing out a review problem and offering a solution

Discussion with NIH staff: Applications often find their way to the wrong referral officer. These cases are usually resolved by discussion of the application content between referral officers. Questions about study section assignments are frequently discussed with SRAs. Questions about an institute assignment may be discussed with the institute staff. The latter is almost always the case when a competing continuation application has a significantly different scientific emphasis than the original application and is a candidate for reassignment to a different institute or when the relevance of an application to an institute's programs has to be confirmed.

What can you do to assist the process? Remember you have toiled long and hard to prepare an application. Do not jeopardize your chances by inadequate attention to the referral process. You may have good reasons for trying to channel your application to a particular NIH institute or study section and if so, do not miss the opportunity. Consider the following:

(a) Enclose a covering letter with the application requesting assignment to a specific institute or study section (three suggestions are allowable), but make sure the request is defensible. If the Referral Office cannot comply, you will receive an explanation. In the case of the institute assignment, familiarize yourself with the program organization and interests of the NIH institutes by referring to Chapter 2 or NIH literature. For information about study section and institute committee review capabilities, refer to Appendixes 4 and 5. In addition, you can obtain committee membership rosters by requesting a copy of *NIH Advisory Committees* from:

Committee Management Office
Building 1, Room 300
Bethesda, MD 20892
(301) 496–2123

A word of caution about the rosters. With the large number of members involved and with approximately one-quarter rotating off a committee each year, it is impossible to keep the roster book current. The date next to each name indicates when the appointment term ends. Also, many of the study sections have subcommittees. For example, the Bacteriology and Mycology study section has two, designated as BM-1 and BM-2 (see Appendix 4). However, the roster book lists the membership of the study section alphabetically without reference to subcommittees. An up-to-date listing of the members of the various subcommittees of a particular study section or institute review committee can be obtained by writing to the Committee Management Office.

(b) Consult with the NIH program staff: The staff member may wish to send a memo to the Referral Office supporting the assignment requests in your covering letter. Such memos usually carry considerable weight.

(c) Application title: Save the exotic, scientific terminology for the body of the proposal! Remember, when the staff starts sorting applications, the title will be read first. Make sure the title reflects a relationship with NIH programs. Simple titles sending clear, instructive messages are preferable, e.g., "Synthesis of Cancer Chemotherapeutic Agents," or "Physiologic Studies of Kidney Transport Mechanisms." Note that both the institute and approximate study section signals are flashing. The latter is especially important to get the application to the right referral officer during the sorting procedures. For competing continuation and supplemental applications, retain the same title as the original application.

(d) Description: This is an important section of the application and should be carefully prepared following closely the instructions printed directly on page 2 of the forms. In all probability it will be the most widely read part of your application! This is not to diminish the importance of the body of the application, but in reality what happens? Logically the referral officer will read this section first to get acquainted with the application and its content. If you have done your job well, that together with your grant history records and biographical data may quickly determine a correct assignment. Next, the application goes to the study section and is mailed to members. They obviously will concentrate on those applications specifically assigned to them for written reviews and probably will scan the remainder of the applications as time permits, focusing again on page 2 to determine what the research is all about. The institute program staff receive copies and in preparation for study section meetings will probably concentrate on page 2 of the application and review the other support you have listed. After the study section meeting, the SRA will use page 2 for a description of your project in preparing the summary statement. The completed summary statements are sent to council members, and again the description of your project will be there for the reading. And this is not the end of the chain! When competing continuation time rolls around or when you submit a supplement or an amended application, the summary statement again appears as a source of background information for the use of study section members. Simply put, pay attention to page 2 and make sure it adequately conveys the requested information and any messages about the institute or study section assignment that you wish to send. But be sure the narrative of the abstract relates directly to the specific aims and research plan of the application.

(e) Be sure your application can be readily identified. If it is in response to an RFA or some other special institute initiative, make sure this is noted on the face page of the application. For example, if you are responding to a Program Announcement, either reference the issue of the NIH Guide for Grants and Contracts or, if it is brief, attach a copy of the PA to a covering letter. Referral officers may be unaware of some Program Announcements because there is usually no expiration date and new ones are constantly being generated.

FINAL PROCESSING

Following institute and study section assignments, the application is sent to the processing unit for final Referral Office action and distribution.

Distribution

The original and six copies of the application submitted by the PI are distributed as follows:

- The original goes to the sponsoring institute to become the first entry in the official grant file.
- One copy is sent to the NIH print shop. About fifty copies of each application, printed by photo offset, are ordered for use by the study section, council, and sponsoring institute.
- One copy is retained in the Referral Office.
- One copy is sent to the Information Systems Branch, DRG, for additional data capture.
- Three copies are sent to the study section office so that the SRA can begin the work-up of the application without print shop delays. A duplicate copy of the official grant file is created for the continuing use of the study section office.

Notification

Approximately six weeks after receiving the application, the DRG will notify you by computer-generated letter of its status. Aside from acknowledging receipt of your application, the letter serves to inform you and your institution of the application number, the sponsoring institute's contact and phone number, study section assignment, and name, address, and phone number of the SRA.

Do not delay in reading the letter to determine if your application is on track and on schedule. If there is a problem, write or call the office of the Chief, Referral Section (see address and phone number below). If you wait too long, the application will have been mailed to reviewers and any requested remedial action becomes more difficult. The result may be postponement to the next review cycle.

Application Number Explanation

In the top right-hand corner of the face page, there are boxes for entry of Referral Office information and decisions. The boxes refer to:

- *Type:* The most commonly used designations are:
  Type 1 New Application
  Type 2 Competing Continuation
  Type 3 Supplement
- *Activity:* There is a PHS code for each grant mechanism. Commonly used ones are R01, R29, P01, K04, and T32.
- *Awarding Unit Code:*

Awarding Unit	Code
NIA	AG
NIAID	AI
NIAMS	AR
NCI	CA
NIDCD	DC
NIDR	DE
NIDDK	DK
NIEHS	ES
NEI	EY
NIGMS	GM
NICHD	HD
NCHGR	HG
NHLBI	HL
NLM	LM
NCNR	NR
NINDS	NS
NCRR	RR
FIC	TW

- *Number:* There are several parts.
  - Serial number: This is a five-digit number.
  - First year of support requested: This is a hyphenated two-digit number which will be -01 for a new application and whatever applies to a specific competing continuation, e.g., -04 or -06, etc.
  - Amended application: The letter A is used, followed by a one-digit number to indicate whether the application is a first or second amendment, e.g., A1 or A2, etc.
  - Supplement: The letter S is used, followed by a one-digit number to

indicate a first or second supplement, e.g., S1 or S2 to a particular grant year.

Examples of application numbers are:

1 RO1 AI 12345–01A2: This is a new, competing regular research grant application assigned to the NIAID and is a second amendment to the original submission.

2 T32 AG 02567–06: This is a competing continuation (renewal) of an institutional training grant, assigned to the NIA, and applying for the sixth and subsequent years of support.

3 PO1 CA 98765–10S1A1: This is a supplemental application to a NCI program project. It is an amendment to a previously unsuccessful first supplement to the tenth year of the project.

INTERNAL CHECKS AND BALANCES

From the print shop, copies of the application are sent to the sponsoring institute and to the study section or review committee office.

In each institute, applications are received in a central location. Based on content, they are referred to the most logical program office, where they can be read by the staff. At this point assignment decisions can be reviewed and challenged if necessary. The emphasis probably will be on the appropriateness of the institute assignment. However, if the staff is aware of review or review group problems, it is quite legitimate to bring these to the attention of the Referral Office. This assignment check is especially desirable early in the process. However, in some cases it may not occur until just prior to a study section meeting due to other staff time constraints.

The SRA of the study section must read the application as soon as preliminary copies are received from the Referral Office. Thus, a valuable assignment check occurs in conjunction with preparing the application for mailing to study section members. The check here will probably include the appropriateness of the study section assignment, application completeness, changes made to amended applications, type 1 versus type 2, and possibly the institute assignment.

Unquestionably, this internal check by the NIH staff helps ferret out many misassignments. However, some do slip through and can cause real problems for applicants. Thus, it is important to note the funding component and review panel assignments in the notification letter.

FINAL COMMENTS

There is constant pressure to keep the mountain of paper flowing. Mistakes do happen! Start your application off on the right foot by understanding the referral process and give it as much attention as it requires. The two key decisions are the study section and institute assignments. If the outcome of the study section review is a low priority score or worse, nothing will help your application get funded. Look over the guidelines for referral to the study sections in your disciplinary or specialty area. If necessary, obtain the most recent study section rosters. Consider exercising your option of requesting a specific study section assignment, especially in the case of a new application. Because of the nature of your research, you might be able to make a legitimate and reasonable case to have your application assigned to any one of several institutes. Familiarize yourself with their program interests and funding ability. In fiscal 1991 the overall NIH success rate for competing research projects R01s was 27.7 percent. However, several of the institutes were able to exceed this rate (see Table 4.3, Chapter 4). After your homework is complete, make your suggestions in a succinct, rational manner in a covering letter.

KEY CONTACT POINTS

Office	Address	Telephone
Chief, Referral Section Special Assistant Assistant Chief Assistant Chief	Room 248, Westwood Bldg. RRB/DRG, NIH Bethesda, MD 20892	(301) 496–7447
Chief, Project Control	Room 253, Westwood Bldg. RRB/DRG, NIH Bethesda, MD 20892	(301) 496–7324

ELECTRONIC SUBMISSION OF APPLICATIONS

There is currently under development a project that will allow the submission of R01 proposals electronically. Some of the goals of the project are to speed application processing time, reduce processing costs, improve data reliability, and improve staff access to applications and data. Procedures are being developed to allow capture of the entire application in the NIH mainframe computer and allow on-line use of data by staff.

Some of the proposed benefits for applicant institutions are a standard, repeatable application preparation procedure; no copying required; rapid (approximately twenty-four hour) notice of application receipt and acceptance; more efficient assistance to PIs; more efficient management of data and content; and the future possibility of an accelerated review cycle.

Some of the proposed benefits for the PHS are elimination of the paper storm; elimination of manual data entry; reduction of application validation and edit time;

reduction in number of applications returned; elimination of application printing delays; improvement in internal and external communications; and better access to data and content.

Field testing of the project is currently underway. For more information, write or call:

The Electronic Grant Operation Project
Division of Research Grants, NIH
Westwood Building, Room 2A05
Bethesda, MD 20892
(301) 402–1464

7

The Peer Review System

The peer review system is an administrative creation first utilized by the NIH over forty years ago. It has enabled the NIH to recruit large numbers of prominent, primarily nonfederal scientists from institutions of higher learning, hospitals, research foundations, and industry within the United States and neighboring countries. This impressive array of expertise is used by the agency to evaluate the scientific merit of grant and contract proposals. It represents a unique partnership between the NIH and the biomedical research community. The scientific expertise contributed by the nation's biomedical researchers would be impossible for the NIH to duplicate with its own staff. On the other hand, the NIH represents an ideal rallying point for the research community for advocating strong, continuing support for biomedical research.

The peer review system is essentially the heart of the scientific decision-making process for the selection of extramural awards, their dollar size, and length of commitment. Thus, a clear understanding of the functioning and staffing of the system is advantageous in many ways in the quest for NIH research support.

The more specific details of nomenclature, scientific coverage, and operations and management of study sections and related review committees are provided in this chapter and the two that follow. Appendixes 4 and 5 list the various scientific review groups, together with the areas of science each evaluates. Advisory councils are discussed in Chapter 10. The essential roles of scientific review groups and advisory councils in the peer review process have been recognized by Congress, which has prescribed their use by law.

DUAL REVIEW OF GRANT APPLICATIONS

Competing grant applications are evaluated by the agency's peer review system using a two-step process. The first level of review is carried out by panels of experts usually organized by scientific discipline and medical specialty, e.g., biochemistry, immunology, pathology, and surgery. Their primary task is to judge scientific and technical merit of proposals and make recommendations to an ICD and its advisory council. These review panels (Table 7.1) are sometimes referred to generically as

TABLE 7.1. Categories of NIH Advisory Committees, FY 1989*

I. Scientific Review Groups		
DRG study sections	1,434 members	(51.1%)
Institute review committees	620 members	(22.1%)
II. Advisory Councils	366 members	(13.0%)
III. Program Advisory Committees and Boards of Scientific Counselors	388 members	(13.8%)
Total	2,808	(100.0%)

*DRG Peer Review Trends 1974–89.

scientific review groups (SRGs) or more commonly as initial review groups (IRGs). Those managed by DRG are referred to as study sections and are responsible for reviewing mostly unsolicited applications of trans-NIH interest. Panels managed by the various NIH institutes are usually referred to as review committees or groups or panels and are responsible for reviewing applications of special program interest. However, in practice in the research community, many of the terms for SRGs are used interchangeably.

The second level of review is conducted by an advisory council or board affiliated with each NIH institute. For each council, Congress has designated the size and the composition of the membership, which is usually a mix of scientific and lay representatives with special expertise or interest related to the mission of the particular institute. The council recommendation is based on the results of the first level of review, program relevance, funding priorities, or other matters of a policy nature.

The law requires a grant application to undergo both levels of peer review in order to be funded. There are two exemptions that permit funding after the first level of review: research grant applications not exceeding $50,000 direct costs per year and fellowship applications.

The purpose of the dual review system is to clearly separate questions of scientific merit from those of a programmatic and budgetary nature. The prevailing theory is that the scientific judgments of study sections are subject to distortion if they are confused with a number of "nonscientific" fiscal and policy matters. Thus, there is a strong feeling that the best interests of science and society are protected by confining the first level of review to assessments of science, and the second level of review to matters of program relevance and funding priorities, in addition to science. The dual review system is summarized in Table 7.2.

PEER REVIEW OF CONTRACT PROPOSALS

Before a Request for Proposals (RFP) is released, the concept and RFP rationale must be approved by an institute ad hoc scientific group, program advisory committee, or the advisory council. Program advisory committees are made up, for the

TABLE 7.2. Dual Review of Grant Applications

First Level of Review

Scientific Review Group

* Evaluates scientific merit
* Rates the quality of acceptable applications
* Recommends budget levels and duration of support
* Does not make funding decisions

Second Level of Review

Council

* Considers review group recommendation
* Evaluates program priorities and relevance
* Advises on funding decisions
* Advises on issues of public policy

most part, of nonfederal, scientific consultants who ensure not only that the concept is sound but that the necessary technology and resources are available to carry out the objective(s) of the RFP.

Proposals received in response to the RFP solicitation are evaluated by a peer review committee, in principle similar to a grant review group but using review criteria tailored to the requirements of the RFP and a different rating procedure.

The second stage of review is conducted by an institute senior staff committee, which usually considers the results of peer review, responsiveness of proposals, proposal budgets, and availability of funds.

OTHER ADVISORY COMMITTEES

There are other segments of the peer review system and types of advisory committees that are less well known but which have a significant impact on the extramural and intramural programs of the NIH.

Institute Program Advisory Committees

Many of the individual institutes have established advisory committees to provide guidance to the staff in the scientific management of their extramural programs. This advice, while not binding, is a significant adjunct to that obtained from other sources, such as institute-sponsored workshops or ad hoc groups. Such committees supplement the role of advisory councils and are able to offer advice in an organized and continuous fashion, with attention focused entirely on specific program or mission issues. Examples of agenda items might be the continuous monitoring and assessment of a specific area of science or disease; identifying gaps in scientific areas in extramural grant and contract portfolios or the converse; selecting and prioritizing ideas for RFAs and RFPs; reviewing the midterm progress of center grant programs; determining the effectiveness of existing grant mechanisms; and assisting in the development of new grant mechanisms. Committee meetings usually are open to the public, but may be closed during the review of progress of funded grants. Members of the scientific community who wish to attend such meetings should contact the staff. A partial list of these committees follows, together with the institute affiliation in parentheses:

- Acquired Immunodeficiency Syndrome Program Advisory Committee (OD/NIH)
- Recombinant DNA Advisory Committee (OD/NIH)
- AIDS Research Advisory Committee (NIAID)
- Dental Research Advisory Committee (NIDR)
- Arteriosclerosis, Hypertension, and Lipid Metabolism Advisory Committee (NHLBI)
- Blood Diseases and Resources Advisory Committee (NHLBI)
- Cardiology Advisory Committee (NHLBI)
- Clinical Applications and Prevention Advisory Committee (NHLBI)
- Pulmonary Diseases Advisory Committee (NHLBI)
- Sickle Cell Disease Advisory Committee (NHLBI)
- Deafness and Other Communication Disorders Program Advisory Committee (NIDCD)
- National Diabetes Advisory Board (NIDDK)
- National Digestive Diseases Advisory Board (NIDDK)
- National Kidney and Urological Diseases Advisory Board (NIDDK)
- Division of Research Grants Advisory Committee (DRG)

Boards of Scientific Counselors

The programs and performance of intramural laboratories, research projects, and investigators are evaluated by boards of scientific counselors. These are peer review committees of nonfederal scientists with expertise in areas of research related to an institute's intramural program. The program of each laboratory and investigator is reviewed at least once every four years. Written reports including recommendations are prepared. Reports are presented at least annually at advisory council meetings. Thus, the boards of scientific counselors serve an important dual function of providing expert scientific advice to the individual institute programs as well as to the NIH about the overall quality of its intramural endeavors.

ORGANIZATION OF NIH SCIENTIFIC REVIEW GROUPS

From the beginning of the extramural programs, the practice has been to maintain a centralized resource at the NIH for the review of grant applications. That responsibility has always resided with an independent NIH component, DRG.

There are several reasons for this administrative arrangement. First, there is the matter of efficiency. The oldest and largest of the grant programs, the R01 program, consists of unsolicited applications that are investigator-initiated and of potential appeal to several institutes. Establishing study sections in each of the various institutes for reviewing such applications would mean a duplication of staff and consultant resources and increased cost. Therefore, the 100 or so study sections continue to be under the jurisdiction of DRG. They review over 20,000 applications per year as a service for most NIH institutes. Second, localizing the review function helps to ensure consistent and uniform standards of review and facilitates monitoring of the system. Another benefit is the ability to develop and train a group of professionals possessing special expertise in peer review procedures. Finally, centralization of review in an independent locale minimizes real or apparent staff conflicts of interest in the review and management of the program. This arrangement fixes responsibility so that review staff is accountable for review and program staff for program decisions.

As the programs grew and their complexity increased, a large number of new grant mechanisms were created tailored to the needs of the individual institutes. It soon became evident that the special nature of these mechanisms, such as multidisciplinary program projects and centers, required that they be reviewed by the institutes rather than in DRG. This led each institute to create a separate review unit within its extramural programs modeled after the larger DRG system in theory and practice. Today there are approximately fifty scientific peer review groups evaluating institute contract proposals and special grant applications. The major difference between the institute-based review units and DRG is the type of mechanisms reviewed. These are summarized in Table 7.3.

MEMBERSHIP OF SCIENTIFIC REVIEW GROUPS

Scientific review groups make up by far the largest category of committee within the NIH peer review system. There are approximately 100 study sections in DRG and fifty review committees in the various institutes. In FY 1989, these committees had 2,054 members. In addition, there are a host of ad hoc consultants, site visitors, and mail reviewers who are called upon for assistance.

Members are drawn from the national pool of scientific talent at research-oriented institutions. Membership is demanding and time-consuming. Therefore, it is truly remarkable that the NIH has been able to attract so many outstanding

TABLE 7.3. Peer Review of NIH Support Mechanisms

DRG	Institutes
Traditional research projects (R01)	Program projects (P01)
FIRST Awards (R29)	Center core grants (P30)
RCDAs (K04)	Specialized center grants (P50)
Postdoctoral fellowships (F32)	Comprehensive center grants (P60)
Senior fellowships (F33)	Institutional fellowships (T32)
SBIR, Phase I (R43)	Special K awards (K07, K08, K11, K12)
SBIR, Phase II (R44)	Conference grants (R13)
AREA (R15)	Responses to RFAs (R01)
Others (see Appendix 4)	Responses to RFPs (N01)
	Others (see Appendix 5)

scientists to serve on these committees. The monetary compensation certainly is not a factor, since the honorarium is $150 per day, and then only for time spent at meetings. All the time spent at home preparing for meetings and writing reports is donated by members. Why then do busy scientists agree to serve? Most find it an educational and stimulating experience to interact with prominent peers to discuss scientific ideas and methodologies. A bonus part of the educational experience is learning from the inside about the administration of the NIH grants program and the personnel responsible for its management. Many scientists feel a civic obligation to repay the agency for the support they receive. Most like to be involved in scientific decisions at a national level, and most consider it prestigious and an honor to serve.

Unfortunately, in recent years, there has been a greater reluctance to serve. One reason for this is undoubtedly due to the workload, which requires an estimated commitment of between thirty and forty-five days per year for homework, travel, and time spent at meetings. Other factors that are probably involved to some extent are a frustration with the low funding rates, raising questions of whether the expenditure of that much time and effort is worthwhile; concern about the review of one's own application, which cannot be reviewed by the study section or committee to which one is appointed; and perhaps some apprehension about being involved in a decision process that may antagonize others in the scientific community working in the same or related research areas.

For most investigators, the decision to serve is straightforward and positive. Those who are unsure or negative should not lose sight of the advantages of service. Before declining, talk to several of your colleagues who have served and have your questions answered by the NIH staff. After many years of observing the peer review system from the inside, two things are quite evident: In general, members of committees derive a great deal of satisfaction and knowledge from service; and, without the assistance of the best scientific expertise, the credibility of the system would be severely challenged to the detriment not only of its achievements to date but also to the thousands of grant applicants who derive benefits from the written evaluations of their research ideas. Fortunately, the response of the scientific community has been very good over the years and is one of the key reasons for the success of the enterprise to date.

Qualifications for Membership

The following criteria are required for selection of members or ad hoc reviewers:

- Demonstrated competence and achievement as an independent investigator
- Mature judgment, which infers fairness, objectivity, and the ability to maintain a balanced perspective
- Commitment to complete work assignments
- Ability to work effectively in a group context
- Personal integrity to assure confidentiality of proposals and discussions

In addition, there are administrative requirements or restrictions placed on the staff in appointing members. A noninclusive list follows:

A person can serve on only one USPHS advisory committee at a given time. However, membership on a committee does not preclude service on an ad hoc basis elsewhere in the system.

A committee can have only one member per institution, except in the case of specified multicampus universities.

The number of federal employees on a committee may not exceed 25 percent of the membership. However, in DRG the limit is one federal employee per study section and in certain areas where the expertise predominates in the VA, two may be permitted.

There must be a one-year lapse in service before an individual can be reappointed to another advisory committee.

Committee appointments are not to exceed four years. The terms of appointment are usually staggered so that approximately one-quarter of the membership retires each year.

Each slate of nominations must include a woman and a member of an ethnic minority group.

Geographic balance must be considered in the appointment of members.

There must be an appropriate balance of experienced and younger members.

Who Is Responsible for Selecting Members?

The most important and key figure in the peer review system is the government official in charge of a study section or review group, the executive secretary. In

April 1991, the title "executive secretary " was changed officially to "scientific review administrator" (SRA). The SRA in charge of each review group has the important responsibility of identifying and nominating members. SRAs must ensure that the panel has the proper scope and depth of expertise to meet the high standards of review expected. Nominations are approved by higher authorities before being finalized. This involves a check of publications, grant records, and seniority.

Sources of Information Available for Assisting Scientific Review Administrators in Nominating Members

- Recommendations from the NIH program staff and other DRG/SRAs
- Review of the individual's grant and contract records
- Suggestions from current or past members or others in the scientific community
- Personal interactions at scientific meetings and service as an ad hoc member or as a member of a site visit team
- Scientific literature
- Consultant files

Selection of the Chairperson

The SRA selects the chairperson with the concurrence of a supervisor. Appointments are usually for the last two years of a four-year term. Basically two criteria are used: (1) Prominence and seniority in the area of science represented by the review group and the respect of its members; and (2) compatibility with the SRA because of the close working relationship that is required.

The chairperson presides over all scientific discussions at meetings and acts as the chief scientific adviser to the SRA.

The NIH Reviewers Reserve

Scientific review administrators have always had the flexibility to invite ad hoc reviewers to supplement expertise, relieve the strain of heavy workloads, and substitute for absent members. The NIH Reviewers Reserve was created to formalize this practice and to insure that ad hoc reviewers meet the same standards and appointment conditions as regular members. The Reserve is made up of retired and former members and other highly qualified scientists not currently serving on NIH committees. Appointments are for nonrenewable terms of up to four years. When serving in an ad hoc capacity, members of the Reserve are accorded the same voting rights and privileges as regular members. Members are free to accept appointments to regular review groups any time they are offered. Responsibility for managing the Reserve for all NIH review groups resides with the DRG.

Members of NIH Advisory Groups

A roster of NIH public advisory groups is published annually. It lists NIH scientific review groups, as well as other advisory committees, together with their functions and names and institutional affiliation of members. If you want to know the possible reviewers of your grant or contract proposal, obtain a copy by contacting:

> **NIH Committee Management Office**
> **Building 1, Room B1–56**
> **Bethesda, MD 20892**
> **(301) 496–2123**

Some Characteristics of DRG Study Section Members

Some of the principal findings from data compiled by DRG (DRG Peer Review Trends) covering the period FY 1979–89, are:

Between the years 1979 and 1989, there was a 71 percent increase in study section membership.

The proportion of members with M.D. degrees declined from 42.2 percent in 1979 to 28.4 percent in 1989.

The average age of members remained at a fairly consistent forty-five.

The number of women more than doubled from 132 (15.8 percent) to 313 (21.8 percent).

Minority representation rose from 4.7 percent (37 members) in 1977 to 16.2 percent (233 members) in 1989. Of the 16.2 percent, the largest minority group was of Asian/Pacific Island origin (11 percent), followed by Hispanic (3.6 percent), black (1.5 percent) and American Indian/Alaskan native (0.1 percent).

The proportion of members employed by institutions of higher education ranged from 84 percent in 1979 to 87 percent in 1989. Those holding the academic rank of full professor declined from 74.1 percent in 1979 to 62.7 percent in 1989. Associate professors rose from 22.7 percent to 31.6 percent and assistant professors rose from 1.8 percent to 2.8 percent.

• About two-thirds of the members had one or more NIH extramural awards in 1986, the last date for which published data are available.

GENERAL COMMENTS

Over the years, the peer review system has been subjected to intense scrutiny by several external and internal high-level committees. In the case of congressional or departmental studies, the conclusions have always been the same: accolades for the system and recommendations strongly endorsing its preservation and protection. In the case of internal studies, there have been a series of recommendations for its improvement, most of which have been implemented.

While the system has been applauded, it has also been widely criticized. A brief summary of some of the reasons cited for its success and some of the criticisms follows. Some of the positive attributes are:

- The rich reservoir of scientific expertise the NIH can draw upon because of the willingness of members of the scientific community to participate
- Scientific decisions and recommendations made by one's peers
- Face-to-face discussions by reviewers of the merits of proposals in the context of a committee meeting. This helps to resolve such matters as those related to differences of opinion on the science, the budget, and the ability of the investigator to conduct the research. It also insures that a variety of views are heard and involved in the decision making.
- The great flexibility of the system. If a review group does not exist or for some reason cannot review a proposal, an ad hoc group can be assembled without too much difficulty.
- The orderly process and well-developed review procedures
- The improvements that have been introduced, such as early release of summary statements, revisions in the rating system (percentiling), and establishment of a formal appeals system
- The management expertise of the NIH staff, which permits smooth functioning and proper monitoring of the system

The system is by no means infallible. Mistakes are made and problems do exist. A major criticism is the extreme conservatism of the reviewers, which does not bode well for unconventional research with high payoff potential or applications without preliminary data. For the most part, this criticism is difficult to refute. Another charge is that the system is elitist and favors investigators from the more prestigious institutions. The data support such perceptions. However, in reality, a significant number of the most scientifically talented individuals are on the faculty of such institutions. In the end, fairness in the system has to be accepted on faith, a concept that leaves many critics unpersuaded.

A related issue is the perception that an "old boy network" exists, wherein members favor proposals from their colleagues and friends and that retiring members name their own successors. There is no way to disprove these notions. These matters must be left to the vigilance of the NIH staff and the objectivity of the vast majority of reviewers. There are, in addition, many other barbs aimed at the system, such as the existence of scientific bias, conflicts of interest, and excessive funding of some investigators. Finally, there is an undercurrent of dissatisfaction, very infrequently vocalized in public, about the performance of some of the NIH review staff. These criticisms relate to the less than laudable quality of many summary statements, inappropriate selection of study section members, and in the case of some, inadequate training before being placed in key positions.

A dramatic increase in the award rates surely would serve to calm the very real and understandable insecurities that exist in the research community. When less than 30 percent of the ROI proposals are funded annually, the result is a significant number of investigators with varying degrees of hostility toward the peer review system.

8

Division of Research Grants
Study Section Review

The Division of Research Grants (DRG) consists of the Director's Office, the Office of Administrative Management, and two branches, the Referral and Review Branch (RRB) and the Information Systems Branch (ISB) (Fig. 8.1). The ISB provides computer and statistical services to the USPHS related to applications and grants. The referral and assignment process and the study sections of NIH are managed by the RRB. The study sections are "regular" or permanent panels that are chartered by the NIH. Other chartered groups are Special Emphasis Panels (SEPs), the members of which are recruited on an ad hoc basis and who serve for one meeting only. Thus, there are eighty-four study sections; sixteen of the study sections have multiple subcommittees. The total number of permanent study sections and subcommittees is 102. In addition, there are seven chartered SEPs. The scientific areas assigned to these panels for review and the types of applications reviewed are listed in Appendix 4.

REFERRAL AND REVIEW BRANCH MANAGEMENT

It is very helpful to know the people in charge of the processing and review of applications. Do not hesitate to ask these individuals for help in resolving concerns and answering questions. The overall supervision of the RRB is the responsibility of the Branch Chief, who also carries the title of Associate Director for Referral and Review of the DRG. Working with the RRB branch chief are three assistants. The Deputy Chief for Review has primary responsibility for the management of the study sections. The Deputy Chief for Referral is in charge of the referral system. The Associate Chief for Review shares review responsibilities and is in charge of a variety of personnel matters such as recruiting, training, and deployment of professional and support personnel.

The regular DRG study sections are organized into seven review sections, each

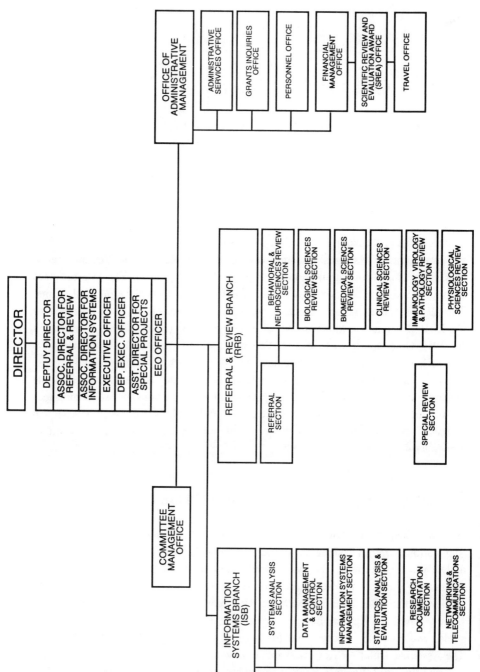

Fig. 8.1. DRG organizational chart.

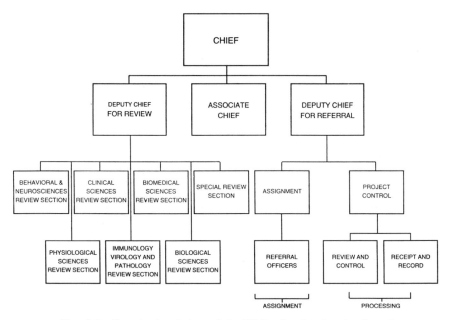

FIG. 8.2. Organizational chart of the DRG referral and review branch.

headed by a section chief who is also an assistant chief of the RRB (Fig. 8.2). These individuals each have an assistant called a lead grants technical assistant. The section chiefs are direct supervisors of the scientific review administrators (SRAs) and support personnel. They are the individuals to turn to if discussions with SRAs are unsatisfactory.

In addition to the permanent study sections, there are SEPs organized and managed in the Special Review Section within RRB. This section has its own staff of twelve SRAs. Other SEPs frequently are organized by SRAs in other review sections to carry out a variety of reviews that cannot be done by a regular study section.

SCIENTIFIC REVIEW ADMINISTRATOR

Most of the SRAs hold a doctorate degree in a field closely related to the science reviewed by their study section. They usually have had previous careers in the research laboratory or the classroom. Some of the key functions of an SRA (Division of Research Grants, National Institutes of Health. 1987. *Handbook for Executive Secretaries*. Bethesda, Md.) are:

- Nominating study section members
- Nominating the chairperson of the study section

- Assigning applications to members of the study section for in-depth review
- Determining if a member is potentially in a conflict of interest situation and taking steps to avoid this type of problem
- Obtaining ad hoc (special) reviewers or opinions on the scientific merit of an application from reviewers outside the membership of the study section
- Arranging the logistics and setting the agenda of the review meeting
- Overseeing the study section reviews, assuring the quality and fairness of the reviews, and compliance with policy and procedures
- Arranging project site visits
- Calculating priority scores and recommended budgets
- Writing summary statements
- Attending advisory council meetings to explain study section recommendations

In most cases, it is quite likely that the SRA is the first person most people in the biomedical research community come into contact with at NIH. In guiding applications through the review process, the SRAs are supposed to serve as the PIs' advocates.

PREREVIEW ACTIVITIES

When the applications arrive in the study section offices, the SRAs, being aware of the referral guidelines for funding components and review groups, check on the referral process. They verify that the applications are suitable for the NIH, whether they have received the correct ICD assignments, and if they have come to the proper study sections. The grants technical assistant, who serves as a chief assistant as well as secretary, logs the applications in, sets up the case files, and starts to collect background information on the applications and the PIs, especially previous applications and summary statements, if they exist. The grants assistants are very knowledgeable and, in many cases, when applicants call the study section office, are able to supply the information sought.

The SRA checks the applications to anticipate the needs of the panel and to assure readiness for review. Such things as the completeness of face page items, key personnel, facilities available, budget items and justifications, information on human subjects, especially the inclusion of women and ethnic minority group members in the study populations, vertebrate animals and potential biohazards, literature citations, and the appendix are examined. In addition, if the application is a competitive continuation or supplement, the SRA will make certain a progress report is included. A review of the scientific sections is done to determine if additional information from the PI is needed. Thus, in the course of the premeeting preparation, a PI may hear from the SRA on a variety of matters. Such communication should be welcomed. It should be realized that the SRA is really acting on behalf of the PI to ensure the best presentation of the application to the study section.

The other important purpose of scrutinizing the science in the application is for the SRA to assign the application to at least two members of the study section for in-depth evaluation at home and discussion of the merits of the proposal at the study section meeting. In addition, at least one member is selected as discussant of the proposal. The SRA becomes knowledgeable about the members' areas of expertise by frequently consulting with them and carefully following their research applica-tion submissions and journal papers.

The SRA may also determine the need for opinions from experts other than study section members or the need for special reviewers to be added to the panel for a particular meeting. In all these matters, the SRA may consult with the panel's chairperson and individual members as necessary.

Applications with background material, such as past summary statements and instructions about the review process, are mailed to the reviewers six to eight weeks before the meeting. Also included in the mailing are statistical data about the priority ratings assigned by individual members and the study section, as a whole, at the previous meeting. This allows the members to evaluate their own rating behavior in comparison with each other and with other study sections, especially those dealing with the same or related areas of science.

This timetable for mailing of applications to members is intended to allow time to complete the assigned in-depth reviews (usually 10–12 per member) and to read the other applications on the agenda. The average workload at a DRG study section meeting is eighty applications. If the reviewers perceive the need for additional information from the PI or an opinion from a scientist outside the panel, they make the request through the SRA. They are asked not to contact the PI directly and, conversely, it is not appropriate for the PI to contact study section members.

If the PI wants to send in new or additional material after the application has been submitted, the SRA should be contacted for advice and instructions. Accep-tance of the materials is at the discretion of the SRA. However, to be sure that the reviewers have an adequate chance to review the new information, and to assure procedural consistency, it should arrive no later than three weeks before the meeting unless specifically requested by the SRA. Thus, it is important to learn the dates of the study section meetings. It is not uncommon for important information to arrive in the study section office after the meeting has finished and therefore not be evaluated in the initial review process.

It is also the responsibility of the SRA to set the agenda for the meeting and arrange the logistics with the aid of the grants assistant. The date usually has been set seven to twelve months earlier. A meeting place and lodging for the members must be secured and NIH program staff made aware of the arrangements.

Meetings take place three times a year. Most will occur in February/March, June, and October/November. Generally the meetings are held in Bethesda; however, some may take place out of town, usually in connection with a national scientific society meeting that most of the members of the study section expect to attend. Dates and locations are published in the *Federal Register* at least fifteen days before the meeting takes place. Also, the study section office can be contacted to learn of the dates. Meetings generally last two to four days, with daily sessions lasting nine to ten hours. The meetings are closed during the review of applications because of the privileged nature of the materials and discussions. Only the staff and reviewers are in attendance.

MEETING AGENDA

The SRA opens the meeting with administrative remarks. These generally include:

- Significant developments at NIH since the last meeting
- Budget and funding information.
- Discussion of rating behavior at the previous meeting
- Housekeeping matters related to the current meeting, including the agenda
- Review of materials not mailed to members, for example, outside opinions and revised or additional application material

The next major item is an explanation of review procedures. Items include:

- Definition of recommendation options. Until recently, the recommendation that a review group could make by majority vote was "approval" (sufficient merit to be worthy of support), "disapproval" (not of sufficient merit to be worthy of support), or "deferral" (no action pending the receipt of additional information). However, Congress, concerned over the increasing approval rate for research grant applications (approximately 65 percent of applications reviewed in 1970 vs. approximately 95 percent in 1990) has suggested that NIH modify its peer review procedures. To provide for a more meaningful distinction between applications that merit funding and those that do not, NIH modified the voting procedures. "Approval" and "disapproval" are no longer used. Review recommendations now focus on two motions:

Deferral The Study Section cannot make a recommendation without additional information. This information may be obtained by mail or by a project site visit.

Not Recommended for Further Consideration The merit of the proposed research is not significant and not substantial, or gravely hazardous or unethical procedures, especially involving human subjects or animal welfare, are proposed. Also falling into this category are supplemental applications (type 3) deemed to be unnecessary or applications in which the study section thinks the named PI will not be responsible for the scientific and technical direction of the project. Applications in this category will not be reviewed by advisory councils.

All Other Applications Based on the review criteria, the strengths and weaknesses of the applications will be discussed and each member will privately rate the application as in the past. Another policy change is that applications which fall into the bottom third of all applications given a priority rating, are no longer automatically reviewed by advisory councils. Exceptions are possible at the initiative of program staff.

- Close scrutiny of the requested budget with attention paid to percent effort in relation to work scope, possible overextension of research staff, justification for equipment and additional personnel in future years, and overlaps with existing support. The recommendation includes justification for modification in amount or duration of the project.
- Explanation of the priority rating system and a request that the full range of ratings be used
- Criteria applied to foreign applications
- Human subjects, vertebrate animals, biohazards
- Explanation of the rules regarding conflict of interest and confidentiality of application materials and the discussions

Conflict of Interest

Review staff and panel members are required to be alert to conflicts of interest, whether real or apparent. A study section or review committee is not permitted to review an application from one of its members. Members do not participate (they absent themselves from the meeting room) in the review of applications from their own organizations. In the case of a multicampus academic institution, e.g., the University of California system, each campus is considered a separate institution. Members absent themselves from the meeting room during the review of applications of close associates, recent students, and scientists with whom they have had long-standing differences that could affect their objectivity. Here, it is perfectly proper for a PI to contact the SRA should there be a concern.

Confidentiality

Review materials and proceedings of review meetings are considered privileged communications and members of review panels are required to leave all review materials with the SRA at the conclusion of a review meeting or site visit. Also, direct communication between members of review groups and applicants is inappropriate and could be detrimental to the review. PIs should not put members who serve on review panels in embarrassing situations by seeking information regarding reviews. All communications are supposed to be handled by the SRA.

Discussion of Individual Applications

Following the administrative remarks and orientation by the SRA, the Chairperson leads the group into the scientific evaluation portion of the meeting. The role of the SRA is to assure that the scientific and technical reviews are fair and thorough, and that all points of view are heard. The SRA must also assure that review policy and procedures are adhered to. It also is important that the SRA follows the reviews in a thoughtful manner so that the resultant summary statements reflect the members' prepared reviews, some of which have to be modified, as well as the relevant ad lib discussions.

Each application is given individual consideration. The Chairperson calls upon the assigned reviewers to provide a description and to discuss the strengths and weaknesses of each proposal. An assigned discussant also presents comments on the merit of the proposed project. In addition, the reviewers scrutinize the organization of the application, the writing, and whether the PI has followed the instructions regarding page limitations, other support, format, etc. Also, it is possible that the impact of the institutional organization and administration and even locale might be discussed. The review criteria that are followed are detailed in chapter 5, "Application Preparation."

The other members of the panel may ask questions of the assigned reviewers during the formal review to clarify points, but the general discussion takes place after the reviewers present their recommendations. It is the responsibility of both the Chairperson and the SRA to encourage discussion of all points of view, especially from those with opposing opinions. Following the discussion, the Chairperson calls for a priority rating to be assigned if it appears from the discussion that there is significant merit to the application. If the proposal does not have significant and substantial merit, a motion may be made that it not be recommended for further consideration. This action is made by majority vote of the panel.

In most cases, the vote is unanimous; however, a split vote for either action can occur. When two or more members dissent, a minority report will appear in the summary statement. If the study section opts for further consideration and provides a priority rating, a budget and period of support must be recommended. The primary reviewers can indicate the approximate rating the application deserves; however, the other members are not bound by this declaration. The review of an individual R01 application usually takes approximately twenty minutes, but could last as long as one hour for more complicated or controversial proposals.

Also present at some meetings are liaison members, usually scientists from the Veterans Administration or the military. They are there to bring information back to their agencies about potentially overlapping programs.

Foreign Applications

Applications from foreign institutions are encouraged and welcomed. However, additional review and funding criteria are applied. Principal investigators should provide information to show whether their proposals involve special talents, resources, populations, or environmental conditions not available in the United States or that would significantly augment existing U.S. resources. Reviewers will determine if similar research is being done domestically and if there is a need for such additional research. In consideration of funding, ICDs look carefully at their program needs and can only fund those foreign applications that fall in the upper 50 percent of priority scores. This does not mean that all that do will be funded. The policy regarding the involvement of women and minorities as part of the study populations in clinical studies must be followed fully. Thus, reviewers will evaluate the PI's material on human subjects similarly to that in applications from domestic institutions, but especially the relevance of foreign populations to U.S. populations, including minorities.

Priority Scores

When one becomes aware of the number of applications reviewed each round by all the review panels and the number that are presented to an individual advisory council, it becomes obvious that many factors have to be considered in arriving at funding decisions. Certainly program relevance and balance are important, but the most persuasive indicators of quality are the written evaluations of the proposals, the accompanying priority scores, and the resultant percentile rankings.

In providing priority ratings, study section members are instructed to rate applications on a scale of 1.0 to 5.0 in 0.1 increments, with 1.0 being the best score. Reviewers are permitted to announce the approximate rating they think the proposal deserves. They are advised further to use the full range of ratings and to be consistent with the following set of prescribed adjectives:

Outstanding	1.0–1.5
Excellent	1.5–2.0
Very Good	2.0–2.5
Good	2.5–3.5
Acceptable	3.5–5.0

Although comparisons sometimes are made between applications, the reviewers are asked to judge each application privately and independently and according to the state of the art in the particular scientific area. Also, they are instructed that ratings should reflect recommended rather than requested budgets. Ratings of each panel member are averaged and multiplied by 100 to arrive at a three-digit priority score.

Until the early 1970s, the "raw" score, the three-digit priority score calculated directly from the reviewers' ratings, was used. However, as funding became tighter and the percentage of awards decreased, it became obvious that there was a diversity of rating behavior among review groups resulting in the observed priority score "creep" (a tendency for better and better scores). Of special concern were cases of different study sections reviewing applications for the same program in a particular institute. For example, there are four immunology study sections (see Appendix 4) and each is likely to review applications for the same program of the NIAID, e.g., immediate hypersensitivity. Because these study sections appear to compete with each other to get their applications funded, comparisons became difficult.

To compensate for differences in scoring standards among review panels, a procedure to normalize scores was developed in the NHLBI and later applied to all priority scores given by DRG study sections. Each study section's raw scores were transformed into a normal distribution with a mean of 250 and a standard deviation of 70. However, normalization was used by only six or seven of the institutes in making funding decisions and was discontinued in early 1980. Dual priority scores (raw plus normalized) on summary statements caused confusion. PIs did not know which score guided funding decisions. Most importantly, Congress started to look at priority score levels in the context of considering appropriations sufficient to fund a "reasonable" number of grants. It too was confused, since some institutes used normalized scores and some did not. In one notable case, an institute's appropriation was shortchanged by several millions because of a mix-up in priority score labeling.

To replace normalization, a procedure to determine the percentile rank of approved applications was developed and quickly gained acceptance in several institutes. Percentiling now has been mandated for all grant-awarding ICDs as the primary indicator of relative scientific merit when applications are being considered for funding. Included are R, U, and fellowship (F32 and F33) applications. P applications, such as the P01, reviewed by DRG special review committees are percentiled, but not P applications (centers) reviewed by ICD panels. Mechanisms also excluded are SBIR (R43 and R44), AREA (R15), training (T), and development (K) awards, which continue to be ranked for potential funding by the three-digit priority scores. Unlike normalization, percentiling does not assume or create a normal distribution of priority scores.

The percentile represents the relative standing or rank of each priority score (along a 100.0 percentile band) among the scores assigned by a particular study section. The lower the numerical value of the priority score or percentile, the better the application. For example, a percentile rank of 25.0 indicates that 25 percent of the applications reviewed by that study section received equal or better scores. In determining the percentile ranking, all applications of a study section from a current plus two previous rounds of meetings (to minimize round-to-round quality variation and to provide stability of larger numbers) are assigned a numerical rank in ascending order of priority score (the best is ranked number 1). The calculation then is p =

100 (K − 0.5)/N: Percentile equals the numerical rank (K) minus 0.5 times 100 divided by the number of reviewed applications (N) in the three rounds. All applications, whether given a priority rating or designated not recommended for further consideration, will be included in the calculation of percentiles.

To qualify for this computation method, a DRG study section must have met for three consecutive rounds and reviewed a cumulative total of at least twenty-five R, P, and U applications.

In the past, changes have been suggested for the rating system, e.g., rating in 0.5 increments, discarding the top (best) and lowest (poorest) ratings, eliminating the rating of a lone "outrider" or disparate score, use of the "olympic" type of scoring, in which each member displays a card indicating the rating given. These suggestions have been tried and the result has been the retention of the current system.

Reasons for Disapproval

A number of studies have been done to determine reasons for the former term "disapproval" of research project grant applications. Several early studies (Allen, 1960, and Wright, 1971), which still hold true today, indicated the following (in decreasing order of frequency):

- The PI does not have adequate experience, training, or both to carry out the proposed research.
- The design is unsound or has serious defects or omissions.
- The approach will not produce useful new knowledge or insight, however sound the approach.
- The experimental approach lacks detail or is too vague.
- The proposal is repetitive of previous work by others or by the applicant.
- The investigator's judgment or knowledge of the state of the art or literature is poor.
- The investigator is not aware of some problems, scientific or administrative, with the proposal or they have not been dealt with adequately.
- The experimental purpose or hypothesis is missing, vague, or diffuse.
- The science is premature or of little importance and warrants, at best, a pilot study.
- The application is superficial, careless, or poorly prepared.

A more recent study (Cuca, 1983) dealing with clinical research applications (research involving human subjects in which a clinician/patient interaction takes place) indicated that the shortcomings of the surveyed proposals were similar to those of all applications.

Deferrals

During the premeeting administrative and scientific review of an application, the SRA and members of the study section try to identify deficiencies in the application.

Answers that can be obtained from the PI prior to the meeting by the submission of reprints, additional information, or simply answers to questions by telephone are sought. Sometimes this is not possible. If the reviewers reach the conclusion at the meeting that there remain serious questions about the proposal and insufficient information to reach a recommendation, deferral will result.

Information will be sought by mail or, if appropriate, by a project site visit (PSV). The purpose of the site visit is to gather information rather than to cross-examine the PI. Also, the purpose is not supposed to be "therapeutic," i.e., to help the PI improve the application.

The visit is preceded by communication between the SRA and the PI. In this exchange, usually by letter, the concerns of the study section are detailed and the logistics of the visit, such as date, place, participants, and agenda, are worked out. The visitors usually include two to four appropriate panel members, ad hoc person(s), if a special problem outside the competence of the study section has been identified, an ICD program staff person, and the SRA. There is generally a breakfast meeting the morning of the visit to decide on the process and strategy of the visit and to determine who will ask specific questions.

PI's are cautioned not to present a seminar that becomes a rehash of what is already in the application, but to be prepared to respond to the study section's concerns. In addressing these concerns, PIs should consider the site visit as a welcome opportunity to highlight the scientific opportunities afforded by the proposed project. If animals are to be used in the research, there may be a specialist in laboratory animal medicine among the visitors who will want to tour the animal facilities. Most site visits for an R01 application generally last no more than six to eight hours.

The PSV team will bring information back to the full study section for action at its next meeting. Under unusual circumstances, e.g., if the PI must do special time-consuming experiments to satisfy the questions, an application can be deferred for two rounds of meetings.

SPECIAL STUDY SECTION

Among the thousands of applications that are received at NIH each year, there are many that present special problems which preclude review in a regular DRG study section. These include those in which the subject matter transcends the review guidelines of several study sections. They may also involve conflict of interest situations, special review requests from advisory councils, special programs such as SBIR, Shared Instrumentation, Biotechnology Resource, some program projects, contracts (rarely), or RFA applications (upon request from an ICD review branch). Many of these applications will be assigned to the Special Review Section of the RRB. Contract and RFA reviews are done mostly by the ICD review panels.

A Special Review Section SRA will organize the review, applying the same general review procedures and standards of conduct that would be used in a regular standing study section. The meeting may take place in Bethesda, at a site convenient to all involved, or in conjunction with a PSV at the applicant institution. The review can also be conducted by a telephone conference call, depending on the nature of the application or the time and circumstances involved. Mail reviews are rarely done except in the case of Conference (R13) applications.

Special Emphasis Panel (SEP)

Because of workload problems, the assignment of applications to the SEPs of the Special Review Section is restricted mostly to the specialized types of applications mentioned above. However, there still are applications that should be assigned to a regular study section, but cannot be for specific reasons. In such a case, an SRA of a regular study section will organize a SEP (formerly designated an ad hoc review [AHR] group) for:

- Members' applications that cannot be assigned to a regular study section
- Conflict of interest situations
- Advisory council- or administratively deferred applications that cannot be assigned to a regular study section
- Workload overflow
- AREA applications
- AIDS applications that cannot be reviewed in the regular AIDS study sections

These reviews are carried out in a manner very similar to those in the Special Review Section. Although there are exceptions, the assigned SRAs usually would be those who are responsible for the reviews of applications of similar subjects in regular study sections. In the case of an SEP, whether reviewing one or several applications, the PI(s) should take advantage of the opportunity to suggest to the SRA the names of individuals whom they do *not* want to review their proposals. Often applicants may want to suggest reviewers, but this is a conflict of interest and is not allowed.

REVIEW OF MEMBERS' APPLICATIONS

An application submitted by a member of a study section cannot be reviewed by the member's own panel. Like any other applicant, the member can suggest not more than three study sections, including an SEP, to review the proposal. And like any other applicant, the member will be accommodated if at all possible. However, if the application cannot be reviewed appropriately by the suggested panels or any other regular study section, it will be assigned to an SEP managed by an SRA of a study section with similar interests in terms of areas of science reviewed, if possible. The SRA of the member's committee cannot manage the review of the application. However, some reviewers from the member's study section may be included (not to exceed 50 percent), but one of these individuals cannot chair the group.

Resigning from a study section so that an application can be assigned to that study section is discouraged. In any case, that particular assignment will not be made by the DRG Referral Office. DRG surveys of new R01 applications from members (a select population considering the criteria for membership) indicate that they do as well as or better than the nonmember R01 population.

These rules and procedures also apply if the PI is a close relative (spouse, parent, or child) of the member, if the member is listed on the budget page for compensation, or if the member is a close professional associate and adviser of the PI and has had considerable input into the preparation of the application and the project. For these reasons, if a PI strongly wishes the application to be reviewed by a particular study section (assuming there is a scientific fit), participation by a member of that study section in the project should be considered very carefully.

POST-MEETING ACTIVITIES

Following the conclusion of the study section meeting, the review staff must calculate priority scores and recommended budgets and input these data along with information on human subjects and vertebrate animals into computer files. This information will appear in a number of reports, one of the most important of which is the summary statement, or "pink sheet," which contains the text explaining the study section's recommendations.

The Summary Statement

The products of the study section's work, the summary statements, are reports that document the panel's evaluations and recommendations for each application reviewed. They are important statements that serve a number of significant purposes. These include use by:

- Advisory councils
- PIs to adjust research protocols or revise unfunded applications
- Program staff to assist in the management of grants
- Grants management staff in negotiating budgets and monitoring adherence to grant policies
- Reviewers, especially when reviewing renewal, revised, or supplemental applications

Formerly, the color of the summary statement for project grant (R01) applications was pink (thus the name "pink sheet"). Other colored papers also were used (yellow for individual fellowships; salmon for program projects; blue for RCDAs; green for institutional training grants). Now, with computer generation of summary statements, all are printed on white paper.

Originally, the summary statement was distributed only to program staffs of ICDs and the advisory councils. If PIs wanted any information about the review, they were sent the essence of the reviews upon request. Now the complete summary statement is sent to the PI on a routine basis. It is constructed by the SRA from the reviewers' preliminary comments and discussions at the study section meeting, and often is quite detailed. Thus, it should be read carefully so that the PI can have the benefit of the reviewers' suggestions as well as a firm basis for revision of the application, if indicated. However, as NIH's workload increases and more expedited reviews are mandated, ways probably will be sought to shorten the summary statement but still maintain its usefulness.

Applicant investigators are able to obtain the reviewers' preliminary comments under the Privacy Act. Since these are destroyed immediately after the summary statement is completed, they should be requested by letter to the SRA within a day or two *after* the study section meeting has taken place. One should remember, however, that some of what is in the preliminary comments may be changed by the discussion at the meeting.

Summary Statement Content

The R01 summary statements consist of the following:

Heading: The recommended action, priority score, percentile ranking, direct costs requested, direct costs recommended, and estimated total costs (direct plus indirect) for each year and the totals, human subject and vertebrate animal information, gender or minority status of human subjects, and indication of any special administrative notes included in the "pink sheet"

Résumé: A brief summary of the objectives of the proposal, its strengths and weaknesses, and reasons for the recommendation

Description: Usually adapted from the PI's abstract. What is proposed, how the work is to be done, and what is hoped will be accomplished.

Critique: An evaluation of the scientific and technical merit of the proposal with details of its strengths and weaknesses

Gender/Minority: Comments regarding the involvement of women and members of minority groups in the study population

Investigator: A description of the key professional personnel and an evaluation of their training, experience, and ability to carry out the proposed project.

Resources and Environment: Does the PI have the resources and is the environment adequate for the work? Are the resources and the environment so special or unique to make support of this proposal a special opportunity?

Budget: The recommended budget with the reasons for specific deletions and modifications in amount or time

Human Subjects/Animal Welfare: If there are concerns (perceived infractions of ethical procedures) regarding the involvement and treatment of humans and animals, these are included in a special note. If there are merely comments (e.g., advice for the PI), these are included in the Critique.

Administrative Note: If the study section wishes to alert the ICD program or grants management staff to some administrative problem, e.g., overlap of the proposed project with other grants or the possibility of duplicate federal funding, this is noted at the end of the summary statement.

Summary statements with priority scores and percentile rankings displayed are sent automatically to all PIs within ten days after they are distributed to the institutes, usually about ten weeks after the study section meeting. One should be aware of the length of time needed to prepare the report. On average, the SRA takes five weeks to complete all the "pink sheets" from the meeting, another two weeks are occupied by typing and proofreading, at least two weeks for reproduction, and then approximately one week for review by program staff. However, under the Privacy Act, PIs may request their "pink sheets" without waiting this long. To assure prompt response to a Privacy Act request, these should be made two to three weeks after the completion of the study section meeting.

OFFICES OF REFERRAL AND REVIEW BRANCH, DRG SECTION CHIEFS

Behavioral and Neurosciences Review Section
RRB, DRG
NIH
Westwood Building, Room 310
Bethesda, MD 20892
(301) 496–7072

Biological Sciences Review Section
Westwood Building, Room 235
(301) 496–0256

Biomedical Sciences Review Section
Westwood Building, Room 336
(301) 496–7071

Clinical Sciences Review Section
Westwood Building, Room 348
(301) 496–7248

Immunology, Virology and Pathology Review Section
Westwood Building, Room A18
(301) 496–0892

Physiological Sciences Review Section
Westwood Building, Room 203
(301) 496–9403

Special Review Section
Westwood Building, Room 2A16
(301) 496–7558

Study sections assigned to each of the review sections are listed in Appendix 4.

9

Institute Review

The study sections in DRG are mistakenly thought by some to comprise the totality of NIH peer review activities. What is often overlooked is the very significant amount of peer review being carried out in the institutes. A few of the mechanisms (program projects, centers, contracts) reviewed in the institutes have received less than favorable acceptance by many in the scientific community because they are perceived to be a less sound way to support research than the R01 award program. Many of the institute reviews involve the most complex grant mechanisms, the most challenging review assignments for staff and reviewers, and result in the commitment of substantial amounts of monies. Approximately 40 percent of NIH funds awarded for competing grant and cooperative agreement in FY 1990 were the result of reviews managed by the institutes. Table 9.1 should serve to highlight the size of the workload.

ORGANIZATION AND MANAGEMENT OF INSTITUTE REVIEW UNITS

Chapter 7 briefly addressed the organization of institute review units. The essential point is that there is a requirement that the review units be organizationally separate from other extramural program activities within an institute. This policy, introduced in the 1970s, initially engendered a great deal of hostility from many program staff members who were used to total responsibility for managing all aspects of their programs, including the review function. A former institute director explained the change in policy at a staff meeting as follows: "It don't look right for the same staff member to write the RFP, choose the members of the review committee, serve as the chairperson of the review committee, collect and calculate the scores, write the summary statements, make the award decisions, and serve as the project officer. So let's get on with it!" While the statement referred to contracts, the message was clear that real or apparent staff conflicts of interest were no longer acceptable. Review staff members were to be responsible for review decisions and program administrators for program decisions.

TABLE 9.1. Applications Requesting NIH Support for FY 1989

Review Location	No. Applications Reviewed	Percent Applications Reviewed
DRG reviews	24,111	82.8
R01 applications	16,735	57.5
T, K, F applications	2,379	8.2
Other applications	4,997	17.1
Institute reviews	5,010	17.2
R01 applications	1,119	3.8
P01 applications	437	1.5
U01 applications	371	1.3
Research centers	360	1.2
K applications	678	2.3
Small grants (R03)	378	1.3
Training grants	560	1.9
Fellowships	329	1.1
Other applications	778	2.7
Total	29,121	100.0*

*Rounded.

Review units in several ICDs are subdivided into branches or sections or both, with each subdivision specializing in the review of a major type of support mechanism or serving a general review function. Still others have an amorphous structure because of the small size of the institute and the review unit. Each unit is staffed with SRAs and grants technical assistants, generally with the same major duties as similar DRG personnel. Each unit has a chief and other supervisory personnel if warranted by its size. In order to facilitate communication among the review units, there is a monthly meeting of all NIH institute review chiefs to discuss current review issues and to share common problems.

The most important similarity between institute- and DRG-conducted reviews are the peer review principles followed. The recommendation options available, the rating system used by members of grant review groups, and the policy requirements are the same, such as rules related to conflict of interest, confidentiality, research involving human subjects, animal welfare, and biohazards. However, there are major differences:

Institute reviews involve for the most part solicited grant applications and contract proposals; almost all DRG reviews involve investigator-initiated applications.
Institute reviews involve a broad array of mechanisms, many of which are designed

for a specific program purpose; the majority of DRG reviews involve fewer mechanisms and are of trans-NIH interest (see Table 7.1, Chapter 7).

Many institute reviews are conducted by ad hoc committees; the majority of DRG reviews are conducted by permanently established study sections.

Institute reviews utilize a number of different review strategies, e.g., triage procedures and project site visits; the majority of DRG reviews follow a similar study section process with very few site visits.

Central NIH monitoring of the review activities of the various institutes, to ensure that uniform and consistent standards are being followed, is difficult. This is in contrast to DRG, where the review activities are relatively easy to monitor since they are located in a single organizational unit.

REVIEW COMMITTEES AND THEIR MEMBERSHIP

Appendix 5 lists the various chartered institute review committees and the types of science they are asked to review. Many of these committees are multidisciplinary in nature, a necessary requirement for the review of certain types of applications, such as program projects. Several of the committees were established to review contracts, most review grant applications, and some are authorized to review both. Nominations for service on these committees are initiated by the SRA of each committee and involve a good deal of consultation with the program staff and other senior institute officials, substantially more than is the case with nominations to DRG study sections. The reasons for this are that staff at all ICD levels are very familiar with the eligible scientists in the communities/constituencies serviced by a particular institute. Additionally, there is more control exercised in the nomination process by supervisory and senior institute officials. However, the selection criteria for membership and the appointment process are virtually identical to the DRG study section procedures previously described. The "invitations to serve" go out under the individual institute director's signature.

Characteristics of Institute Review Group Members*

The number of institute review group members with M.D. and M.D./Ph.D. degrees was 274 or 44.2 percent of the total (620) in FY 1989. This represents a decline from FY 1979, when the numbers were 297 or 52.7 percent of a total of 564 members. In FY 1989, the percent of study section members with similar degrees was 28.4.

---

*DRG Peer Review Trends, 1979–1989.

Of the total number of members in FY 1989, 83.6 percent or 518 were employees of institutions of higher education. The academic rank of these members was: professor, 352 or 68 percent; associate professor 119 or 23 percent; assistant professor, 31 or 6 percent; and instructor/other, 16 or 3 percent.

The number of women members in FY 1989 was 157 or 25.3 percent of the total. In FY 1979, comparable numbers were 138 and 24.5 percent.

The last published data for minority members was in FY 1986. Minority representation was 146 members or 23.1 percent of the total. Of the 23.1 percent the race/ethnic origin breakdown was: Asian/Pacific Islanders, 62 or 9.8 percent; Hispanic, 34 or 5.4 percent; black, 48 or 7.6 percent; and American Indian/Alaskan, 2 or 0.3 percent.

Other characteristics, with comparisons to council and study section membership, are included in Chapter 10.

REVIEW OF CONTRACTS

There was a time when the review of contracts often was a painful experience for staff and reviewers. Many contract review meetings began with a lively discussion of the demerits of the RFP instead of the merits of the contract proposals. The chances of that happening today are rare. Following the policies introduced in the 1970s, there has been a dramatic improvement in the review of contracts. Peer review of the RFP concept and a tightening of the review process have been the major reasons. There also has been greater emphasis in most institutes on supporting research via grants or cooperative agreements rather than contracts whenever possible.

The review procedures for contracts are the most specific of any of the support mechanisms. The review criteria are published in the RFP together with the weighted value to be assigned to each criterion in arriving at an overall rating score (usually the maximum is 100). If no standing review committee exists to review the responses to an RFP, reviewers with the requisite expertise are recruited by an SRA to form an ad hoc committee. Such committees have a highly desirable concentration of expertise, which usually results in a very thorough review.

The agenda and operations of the review committee are similar to those of a grant review committee, with two exceptions: (1) time is allocated on the agenda for a program staff member to discuss the background information and to answer any questions the reviewers may have about the RFP; and (2) the review procedures differ in that the recommendation options are acceptable and unacceptable; and each proposal must be rated on the basis of the weighted numbers associated with each review criterion. Summary statements are prepared for each proposal in a format that presents the strengths and weaknesses for each of the review criteria.

REVIEW OF RESPONSES TO AN RFA

The growing number of RFAs issued has resulted in an increased number of applications added to the workloads of already burdened ICD review staff members. This was a major reason for initiating a triage policy with regard to RFAs. Another reason is the limited time available to conduct reviews, exacerbated by the expedited review requirements for AIDS applications, and other special cases that arise from time to time.

Triage is defined by NIH as "an initial screening by a scientific peer review group of applications according to their relative level of competitiveness, with the intent to eliminate the noncompetitive applications from further consideration." Some of the rules governing the triage policy follow:

The RFA must announce that a triage procedure may be used.

The decision to conduct triage resides with the review staff. It is based on factors such as the number of applications received relative to the available RFA funds; time available to review applications and process awards; and personnel available to carry out the review.

The triage peer review group consists of no less than five members, to include, if possible, the chairperson and other selected members of the review committee recruited to review all responses to the RFA. It is in essence a subcommittee of the review committee.

The triage group rates each application as competitive or noncompetitive in terms of the review criteria.

The SRA chooses the particular type of triage review, such as a formal meeting, either separate or in conjunction with the review committee meeting; teleconference; or mail review.

The noncompetitive applications are not reviewed further. A one-page summary statement is prepared and includes a brief, one-paragraph explanation for the action. The summary statement is sent to the PI shortly after the triage procedure has been completed.

The competitive applications are subjected to a comprehensive review by the full review committee and recommendations prepared in the form of the usual summary statement for consideration by an advisory council.

Provided a similar grant mechanism is available, noncompetitive applications may be submitted as investigator-initiated applications.

The review process is relatively straightforward for R01-type responses to an RFA. If no standing review committee exists to review the responses to an RFA, the SRA will form an ad hoc committee. Again, such a committee should have a highly desirable concentration of expertise, which usually results in a very thorough review. The agenda and operations of the review committee are similar to those of other grant review committees, with perhaps one exception: Time is set aside on the agenda for a program staff member to present background information and to answer questions from the reviewers about the RFA.

REVIEW OF INSTITUTIONAL TRAINING GRANTS

Reviews are conducted by multidisciplinary review committees. The review criteria are:

- Training record for the program and preceptors in terms of the rate at which former trainees establish independent, productive careers
- Training record in terms of the success of former trainees in obtaining individual awards such as fellowships, career awards, and research grants
- Objectives, design, and direction of the research training program
- Caliber of preceptors including successful competition for research support
- Training environment, including institutional commitment, quality of the facilities, and the availibility of research support
- Recruitment and selection plans for appointees and the availibility of high quality candidates
- Record of the program in retaining health-professional postdoctoral trainees for at least two years
- When appropriate, the concomitant training of health-professional postdoctorates (e.g., M.D., D.O., D.D.S.) with basic science postdoctorates (e.g., Ph.D., Sci.D.) will receive special consideration

REVIEW OF PROGRAM PROJECTS AND CENTERS

There is no one method prescribed for the review of these large grants. Thus, some institutes use an initial, two-step review process that includes evaluation of the application by a site visit team and a recommendation by a multidisciplinary review committee. Other institutes consider the two-step process redundant and prefer review solely by a site visit team with its recommendations going directly to a council. Still others use a committee review with infrequent site visits. Some institutes use RFAs to solicit applications for program projects and centers and thus may choose to use a triage process followed by a complete review of competitive proposals by site visit groups or committees.

Recent notices in the *NIH Guide for Grants and Contracts* are indicative of changes in the review process for program projects either being implemented or contemplated. The following appeared in the *NIH Guide* (Vol. 20, No. 18, May 3, 1991):

Effective for the June 1, 1991 receipt date, program project (P01) applications assigned to the National Institute of Child Health and Human Development (NICHD) will no longer be routinely site-visited. These applications will be considered by the relevant Initial Review Group (IRG) without interaction with the applicant. The IRG will have the option of deferring an application for a site visit, although this will be the exception rather than standard practice.

As a result of this change, NICHD P01 applicants must ensure that the description of the proposed research for each component project/core facility is thorough and complete (not to exceed 20 pages*), permitting direct evaluation by the reviewers.

Unless otherwise indicated, NICHD Center Core (P30) Grant and Specialized Center (P50) Grant applications will continue to receive site visits as a part of the review process.

The NHLBI has been using a project site visit (PSV) and review by a standing, program project committee to evaluate its program project applications. It recently published the following notice in the *NIH Guide* (Vol. 20, No. 12, March 22, 1991):

Effective with the receipt of applications due June 1, 1991 and October 1, 1991, new and amended new competitive program project applications assigned to the National Heart, Lung, and Blood Institute (NHLBI) will be reviewed on a schedule longer than has been the custom in the past. This is necessary in order to carry out the usual NHLBI peer review process for program project grant applications at a time when the number of applications has greatly increased. These applications will be reviewed by the NHLBI review branch in as timely a manner as is practicable.

The submission of many program project grant applications in excess of the usual workload has already necessitated the delay in review of many applications and has placed a significant burden on review staff, reviewers, and scheduling. The increased percentage of amended applications has contributed to this problem.

The nature of the program project grant has evolved greatly since its inception in the early 1960s. Because of the recent circumstances, the NHLBI is taking the opportunity in the next 9 months to examine the program project grant mechanism. To this end, two NHLBI staff committees are being established to revise program project guidelines and review procedures. The National Heart, Lung, and Blood Advisory Council and extramural scientists will be part of this process. It is currently expected that new program guidelines and review procedures will be presented to the Council in October 1991 with implementation for the February 1, 1992 deadline.

THE PROJECT SITE VISIT (PSV)

While the PSV is used infrequently in the case of R01 study section reviews (a fraction of 1 percent are site visited), it has been an essential element in the review of program projects and center applications because of their complexity and the

*The page limitation is now increased to 25 pages.

large investment of monies involved. However, change is in the wind; undoubtedly the site visit will be used more judiciously in the future instead of being an automatic part of the review process. Whatever the future holds, a detailed description of a program project PSV that follows may be instructive for those groups involved in such a review event. The information could prove useful in planning for center site visits such as P50 applications, which are similar to program projects, as well as site visits for other types of applications.

The Important Preliminaries

Before writing an application, contact the program and review staff for advice and guidance. You can obtain insights into such matters as the level of interest, restrictions on the level of support that can be requested, the review process, and instructions for preparing an application. Be sure to become familiar with the review criteria used to evaluate program project applications.

Write a well-organized, complete application. Remember that the page limitations described in the PHS 398 instructions or the RFA apply to each component of the program project application and not to the application as a whole. Obtain any supplementary instructional material or brochures that an institute may have available for applicants. Do not count on preparing an incomplete application with the idea of filling in the details at a site visit. That opportunity may never come!

Once you have prepared a draft of the application, ask the program and review staff of the institute to comment on its content, as discussed in Chapter 11. An ideal situation is to have the institute staff visit your institution to discuss the program and the application. An alternative is to arrange for some of the key participants to travel to Bethesda to discuss the application with the staff. In the case of RFAs or during particularly busy times, it may not be possible for the staff to offer the advice or services you desire. However, it does not hurt to try.

The Planning Stage

It is important to establish a good rapport with the SRA, who is one of two key individuals in the site visit process; the other is the Chairperson of the site visit team. There will be a number of issues to discuss, and mutual cooperation will not only facilitate the review but will also alleviate some of the anxiety that is usually associated with site visits. A good way to start is to ask the SRA if there is any way you can help with the arrangements for the site visit at your end, such as suggesting convenient hotels, restaurants, and transportation. But no matter how well you get along with the SRA, do not lose sight of the responsibilities that confront you in carefully planning and attending to the many details associated with such visits.

One of the first things that has to be decided is a suitable date, which is usually subject to negotiation. You will be given the general time period for site visits and asked to come up with dates convenient to you and your team. Be reasonable and offer several choices well within prescribed limits. Make sure your dates do not coincide with holidays or any prominent scientific meetings in your field, which would make the recruitment of reviewers difficult.

Once a date has been agreed upon, the SRA will be free to begin recruiting site visitors. Before the SRA does so, you will probably be asked if you have any concerns about potential reviewers. If you do, be sure to raise them at the outset, because it is most unlikely that the SRA will be willing to disinvite reviewers after the review team is in place. There are several things to keep in mind pertaining to your input on this matter: (1) if there are individuals whom you feel would not be objective as site visit reviewers, bring their names to the attention of the SRA, but be prepared to provide reasons for your objection in each case. The chances are good that your exclusion requests will be honored; (2) the SRA is not supposed to accept the names of potential reviewers from applicants. Once names are volunteered, they are likely to be rejected as site visit participants; (3) if you are concerned about the proper mix of expertise on the site visit team, there is nothing to prohibit you from reviewing with the SRA the major areas of science involved in the application—but do it tactfully; and (4) if your program has outside consultants serving on an advisory group or in some other capacity, the SRA will undoubtedly note this in reading the application. However, it would be well to point this out in case it has been overlooked; it could prove helpful to the SRA in knowing not to consider such individuals as potential reviewers.

An early requirement for the site visit is the preparation of a suitable agenda. In considering how best to structure the agenda, several key points should be kept in mind. The reviewers will receive a copy of the application well before the site visit. It is valid to assume they will have read it and, therefore, there is no need to spend the limited, valuable time available for the visit re-presenting all the material in the application. This is strategically unwise in that it will bore the visitors and markedly reduce the time for questions and answers after each of the scientific presentations. Adequate time for interaction of reviewers with investigators is critically important to insure that the site visitors leave with a more complete understanding of the program than can possibly be gleaned from the application.

Generally, the agenda should be designed to cover the program in one day; an 8 A.M. to 3 or 4 P.M. time period should be sufficient and not overburden the reviewers, who still will have much to do before their day ends.

Usually the SRA will assist you with the agenda, either by providing some written guidelines or by making verbal suggestions. The following are some general rules of thumb to consider in preparing an agenda for a program project or center with up to ten components.

- Allot the first ten minutes for one appropriate official (dean, department chairperson, etc.) to speak about institutional support, policies, administration or whatever is most relevant.

- Allot about thirty minutes for a summary presentation of the program by the Program Director.
- Schedule about twenty or thirty minutes for each project and core, with no more than one-third to one-half of the time for formal remarks. Try to keep the presentation order the same as in the application to make it easier for the reviewers to follow.
- Allow for two ten-minute breaks, one in the morning and one in the afternoon.
- Allow forty-five minutes for lunch. A cold lunch served in the same conference room as the site visit meeting preserves valuable time.
- Include two ten- to fifteen-minute executive sessions to allow the reviewers to exchange notes and to determine what questions still remain to be answered. An appropriate time for one session is right before lunch and the other at the conclusion of the scientific presentations and before a final meeting with the program director.
- A final session with the Program Director should be included.
- A tour of the facilities may or may not be necessary. If it is necessary, try to schedule a tour at a time which is least disruptive to the smooth flow of scientific presentations, such as right before or after lunch or at a time suggested by the SRA.

The agenda will be carefully reviewed by the SRA. Once there is agreement on the schedule, it is unlikely to be changed by the site visit team except in some minor way.

Another important part of the planning process is to hold a rehearsal(s) with all members of the research team present. It is essential that members become familiar with the overall goals of the program, its administrative structure, the different scientific projects and cores, and how they are supposed to interact or collaborate. Make sure that each key participant has read the application. Unless the team is thoroughly briefed, embarrassments can occur at the site visit. The reviewers' questions and informal interactions with team members are bound to uncover any lack of knowledge of the program. The presenters should be the leaders of each project and core. Each should be admonished not to get into long-winded scientific discourses or seminar-type presentations and not to reiterate material already well presented in the application. Instead, a few simple slides might be in order that emphasize the aims of the research, experimental procedures that may require some elaboration, and projected plans for the five-year project period. Once there is agreement about presentations and their general format, audiovisual aids and equipment, and a discussion of the program and the visit, a more formal run-through of the program should occur shortly before the visit. If knowledgeable colleagues who are not participants are available, it might be beneficial to invite them and get their reaction to the presentations.

Before the visit, the SRA will send out the names of the site visitors. It is obviously beneficial for the program participants to become familiar with the reviewers' research interests and their relevant publications.

A copy of the application, or significant sections, should be sent to the institutional official who will address the site visit team. Also, it is a good idea to follow up with a personal briefing of this individual, emphasizing the goals of the program, the organization of the program, including the departments and individuals involved, the administrative structure of the program, including provisions for monitoring and decision making, any unusual budget requests and the justification offered, institutional resources involved or ready to be committed, any prior collaborative history (as would be the case for a renewal), and background information about how the program evolved. Even though this presentation is to be brief, the presenter will feel and appear much more knowledgeable with this information in mind.

The SRA will undoubtedly let you know about the need for reprints, additional budget justifications, explanations about other support, and other supporting materials. At your end, it is highly advisable to identify any necessary changes to the application early on and send them to the SRA so that the information can be mailed to the reviewers well in advance of the visit.

Finally, be sure to prepare a map and very specific instructions to guide the review team in getting from the hotel to the conference room. The site visit may get off to a rocky start with a group of reviewers lost somewhere in a large complex.

The Presite Visit Meeting

The meeting of reviewers the night before a site visit serves several important purposes. The SRA has an opportunity to properly orient the group about the review ground rules that apply to program projects and to site visit teams. The Chairperson and the reviewers have an opportunity to adjust their review and writing assignments. A preliminary roundtable discussion of the application highlights the questions that need to be asked and other initial impressions of the program. The meeting has the added advantage of allowing reviewers to get better acquainted and to permit the Chairperson to review any additional procedures that should be followed. The agenda and plans for the next day are reviewed. If any additional information is required or if there are any minor changes in the agenda, such as including a brief tour of facilities, the SRA will be asked to contact the Program Director after the meeting. If the SRA has not alerted you to this possibility, volunteer your phone number and your willingness to accept a late call.

One thing that is important to avoid is to greet reviewers with last-minute revisions of the application. They arrive at the hotel tired but willing to sit through a presite visit meeting. They will not appreciate having to review new material before going to bed and may wonder how well organized you are, especially if the revisions are extensive. There is also the possibility they may refuse to review the new material, with good cause, because of the insufficient time available to do so.

The Onsite Visit Meeting

In considering a suitable place to hold a site visit meeting, choose a conference room of sufficient size to assure reviewer comfort. There should be a conference table that not only provides ample seating room for the visitors but adequate space for note taking. Name tags for visitors and program participants, pads and pencils for reviewers, a nearby telephone, a blackboard, and a coffee pot are little conveniences that will be appreciated.

The Program Director should make sure the meeting gets started on time. After introductions and brief, informative remarks by an institutional official, a well-organized, lucid presentation by the program director will serve to start the scientific proceedings off on the right track. This an ideal time to describe the goals and all facets of the organization and administration of the program. A noninclusive list of items to consider highlighting are: the significance and importance of the research theme; major accomplishments during the prior project period in the case of a renewal; persuasive reasons for supporting a program rather than individual projects; the organization of the program, with a brief reference to the objectives of each project and core and why each is an essential component of the program; the interactive nature of the projects and cores; if clinical studies are involved, plans for inclusion of women and minorities should be mentioned and elaborated upon in the individual project or core presentations; the caliber of the senior investigators and support staff and any history of previous collaborations; program priorities and plans for a five-year period; significant arrangements with other departments or institutional components; institutional support and any cost-sharing items; the available facilities and any unique aspects of the research, equipment, or resources; how the activities will be coordinated and managed; the role of any advisory committee, collaborators, or other advisers; and any aspects of the budget that warrant special mention. Some of the items might not be relevant and others more appropriate, depending on the program. However, these are the types of issues to be touched on in an opening presentation that sets the stage for what follows. The presentation should be approximately twenty to thirty minutes in duration and include a few slides to emphasize the major points you wish the reviewers to remember about the overall program. Handouts may also be useful, but be careful not to inundate the reviewers with paper.

For the balance of the individual project and core presentations, the Program Director should make every attempt to do the following:

- Take notes of questions that may not have been adequately answered or issues to be brought up at the final meeting with the site visitors

- If a question addressed to a presenter is better answered by a close collaborator, try to bring this about either by quietly motioning to the individual to raise a hand or by calling on the individual to speak. However, it is obviously not wise to embarrass the presenter, so good judgment and timing are important.
- Assist the chairperson in keeping the visit on schedule.
- Make arrangements for the visiting fiscal consultant and/or grants management specialist to meet with an institutional business official(s) at the start of the individual project and core presentations.
- Hold an informal meeting with program participants while the site visitors are in their executive session prior to lunch. This is a good time for participants to compare notes and to identify areas that might require further discussion with reviewers.

Arrangements for lunch should be discussed with the SRA. The site visitors may wish to have a private lunch. However, it is best to encourage a cold sandwich-type lunch in the conference room with program participants present. This encourages informal scientific discussion with reviewers and can serve as an extension of the morning presentations. The advantages of the conference room setting are the presence of a blackboard, pencil and paper, the application and reprints, and the proper ambience for reviewer–investigator interactions, all of which would not be present in a cafeteria.

Infrequently at a site visit, a reviewer may become overzealous or abrasive. The best way to handle the situation is to keep calm even though your instincts urge other actions. At an appropriate time during the proceedings, such as the coffee or lunch break, quietly discuss the matter with the SRA. The SRA will either talk to the reviewer directly or ask the Chairperson to do so.

The final meeting of the Program Director and site visitors is an excellent opportunity to not only amplify on any of the problem areas that your notes indicate developed during the presentations but also to briefly extol the virtues of the program again. The reviewers have now heard all the presentations and met all the participants, and in this context you have an opportunity to add some additional thoughts on why the program is worth supporting, your commitment to the program, and so forth. As long as it is not overstated, any information that would enhance the reviewers' impression of your leadership ability and the importance of the program might be helpful to your case. Finally, at the end of the discussion, it does not hurt to thank the reviewers for coming, for being attentive, and for being fair in obtaining the information they need.

The Postsite Visit Meeting

The session usually begins back at the hotel with the SRA explaining the review procedures to be followed. In the case of program projects and related types of centers, the reviewers probably will be addressing the following criteria:

For Projects and Core Units

- The scientific merit of each research project and its relation to the central theme
- The technical merit and justification for each core unit
- Accomplishments of projects and cores in a renewal or supplemental application
- Qualifications, experience, and commitment of the investigators to the program
- Appropriateness of the budget for the projects and core units
- Adequacy of the protection of human subjects, animals, and the environment and in the case of study populations the inclusion of women and minorities

For the Program as an Integrated Effort

- The significance and importance of the central theme and program goals
- The justification for a cooperative team effort
- The multidisciplinary scope of the program and the interrelation of the projects and cores
- The leadership ability, scientific stature, and time commitment of the Program Director
- The participation of a sufficient number of experienced investigators
- The quality of the academic and physical environment, such as space, equipment, patients, and interaction with other scientists
- The arrangements for quality control, allocation of funds, internal communication, and day-to-day management of the program
- The institutional commitment to the program
- The appropriateness of the program budget

After the review instructions to the site visit team, the Chairperson will operate the meeting similar to a study section. Each project and core will be discussed individually and recommendations voted upon. The attributes of the program as a whole will be discussed and a recommendation made. At this point the visitors will adjourn to write their reports and a time will be set to reconvene to read and modify the written material to be included in the site visit report or summary statement.

GENERAL COMMENTS

Council review aside, the NIH peer review system is not a homogeneous entity. It can be viewed as consisting of two major parts: (1) the well-known study sections located in DRG, a central organizational entity with no program or funding responsibilities; and (2) a network of review units located in each of the institutes, which do have program and funding responsibilities. The major relationship between the two parts consists of the fundamentally similar review policies and procedures that must be followed no matter where the review is conducted. The DRG system is operated with strict separation of review and program functions and unquestioned support by the Office of the NIH Director. On the other hand, the success of an institute review unit is directly related to the attitude and support of the institute director in furnishing adequate resources and keeping overly aggressive program officials in check, both of which do not exist in an acceptable manner across the board. However, it is fair to say that more cooperation and coordination between review and program staff is required at the institute level because of the special nature of the mechanisms involved.

There appears to have been substantial improvement in institute-based reviews over the last fifteen years or so. Many of these reviews are difficult, sensitive, and require a good deal of staff expertise. They also involve mechanisms that some in the scientific community look upon with a jaundiced eye. While it is difficult to change these attitudes, it does increase the pressure to conduct reviews in the most professional manner possible. Of all the mechanisms reviewed in the institutes,

ICD Scientific Review Chiefs

ICD	Address	Telephone
FIC	Building 31, Room B2C39	(301) 496–1653
NCI (Grants)	Westwood Bldg., Room 821	(301) 496–7929
NCI (Contracts)	Westwood Bldg., Room 803	(301) 496–7903
NCI (Logistics)	Westwood Bldg., Room 850	(301) 496–7173
NCHGR	Building 38A, Room 606	(301) 402–0838
NCNR	Building 31, Room 5B10	(301) 496–0472
NCRR	Westwood Bldg. Room 8A16	(301) 402–0314
NEI	Building 31, Room 6A06	(301) 496–5561
NHLBI	Westwood Bldg., Room 557A	(301) 496–7919
NIA	Gateway Building, Room 2C212	(301) 496–9666
NIAID	Solar Bldg., Room 4C19	(301) 496–0123
NIAMS	Westwood Bldg., Room 5A05A	(301) 496–0754
NICHD	Executive Plaza North, Room 520	(301) 496–1485
NIDCD	Executive Plaza South, Room 400	(301) 496–8683
NIDR	Westwood Bldg., Room 519	(301) 496–7658
NIDDK	Westwood Bldg., Room 603	(301) 496–7083
NIEHS	Building 3, Room 310A P.O. Box 12233 Research Triangle Park, NC 27709	(919) 629–1442
NIGMS	Westwood Bldg., Room 9A18	(301) 496–7585
NINDS	Federal Bldg., Room 9C10A	(301) 496–9223
NLM	Building 38A, Room 5S522	(301) 496–4221

program projects and centers require the most time, delicate handling, and skill. The task is not made easier by the absence of uniform NIH review procedures related to site visits, committee reviews, combinations of the two, and different rating methods. With the increased workloads on the review units, it is highly probable that new, more efficient procedures will gradually evolve.

Institute-based reviews have increased in impact and importance over the years and this trend seems to be continuing with the release of greater numbers of RFAs and the many new grant mechanisms being developed. The data appear to bear this out: The ratio of applications reviewed by the DRG compared to the institutes is approximately 5 to 1, but in terms of dollars awarded, the ratio is more like 3 to 2.

The accompanying chart (p. 128) lists addresses and telephone numbers of ICD Review Chiefs.

10

National Advisory Councils

Historically, national advisory councils were the first on the peer review scene. In 1937, Congress created the National Cancer Institute (NCI), along with an advisory council, and authorized the support of research and research training. With the passage of the Public Health Service Act in 1944, the NCI became part of NIH and a National Advisory Health Council was directed to provide support for other areas of biomedical research. After World War II, the NIH inherited a variety of research activities supported by other agencies. The National Advisory Health Council felt the need for scientific assistance in the review of grant applications. In 1946, NIH created the Office of Research Grants, which eventually became the DRG of today, and twenty-one study sections to help the National Advisory Health Council carry out its mandate to make grant awards. This *briefly* is how it all began and may help to place in perspective the origin of national advisory councils, study sections, and other similar scientific review groups.

Over the years, between congressional legislation and reorganizations of the health activities within the DHHS, the NIH grew from the original NCI to the present eighteen components authorized to award extramural grants and contracts, each with an advisory council/board.

FUNCTIONS AND RESPONSIBILITIES
OF AN ADVISORY COUNCIL

An advisory council is analogous to a board of directors. In this case, the available experience and expertise is utilized to advise on program activities, priorities, policies, procedures, and national research and health issues. Institutes use councils in a variety of ways. However, there are fundamental responsibilities that are common to all. Councils are required to:

Review grant applications and make recommendations based on scientific merit and program considerations (This is the second stage of the peer review process.)
Advise the Secretary, DHHS, Director, NIH, and the relevant institute director on matters related to the institute's programs and mission

Prepare an annual report for the Secretary, DHHS. In the case of the NCI and the NHLBI, the report is prepared for the President, Congress, and the secretary. Reports usually include a description of progress made toward achieving the goals of the institute's mission during the preceding fiscal year, future needs, and resource requirements.

An institute can involve advisory councils in numerous other matters, some of which are required by NIH. A few examples are provided below; some will be elaborated upon later.

- Review of extramural and intramural program activities
- Concept clearance for RFPs
- Establishing priorities for new program initiatives
- Approval of RFAs and PAs
- Development of new grant mechanisms
- Reexamination of existing mechanisms
- Review procedures for grant mechanisms such as program projects
- Planning, cost, initiation, and progress of large clinical trials

ADVISORY COUNCIL COMPOSITION

The composition of advisory councils is prescribed by law. The membership ranges from ten members for the NLM Board of Regents to eighteen for four of the institutes. Appointment of ex-officio members is required and this type of membership ranges from two for most institutes to eleven for the National Cancer Advisory Board. Ex-officio members are representatives of other government agencies and serve in a liaison capacity to insure an efficient and timely back-and-forth flow of information.

The majority of members must have expertise in medical and scientific areas related to the mission of the particular institute. However, one-third of the membership must represent the public interest and are usually prominent lay individuals with a special interest in the areas represented by an institute's mission.

The Chairperson of an advisory council is also specified in the law. For most institutes it is the Director, NIH, but in practice the director of the individual institute presides. In the case of the NLM, the Board of Regents elects a chairperson. For NCI, a presidential appointee serves as the Chairperson.

Qualifications for Membership

Scientific members are usually senior biomedical researchers who are recognized experts and leaders in their fields. They must be knowledgeable in areas related to the mission of the institute, have an appreciation of the requirements of a national biomedical research effort, and an appreciation of the health needs of the American people. Besides scientific expertise and research accomplishments, other ideal attributes are an awareness of the functioning of the peer review system, good judgment, an ability to work well in group situations and with the staff, and a commitment to spend the time and effort required.

Public members are usually well-recognized individuals for their achievements in education, law, public health, entertainment, business, philanthropy, community affairs, and so forth, who have an interest in health issues related to the mission of an institute.

Other criteria applied to the selection process include:

- A proper mix of representation from medical specialties and scientific disciplines suitable to cover the range of science involved in an institute's programs and mission
- Adequate representation of women and minorities
- Adequate geographic distribution
- Only one member can be appointed per institution.
- Members cannot serve concurrently on more than one DHHS advisory committee.
- A one-year interval is usually required between successive terms of service on a council.
- Appointments are usually for staggered, four-year terms, with the exception of members of the National Advisory Cancer Board, who are appointed for six-year terms.

Selection of Members

Nominations are initiated by the director of an institute, and sent through the Director, NIH, to the Office of the Secretary, DHHS. The secretary is empowered by the Public Health Service Act to appoint members to advisory councils. The exception is the National Cancer Board, which requires a presidential appointment. The nomination process requires both a "principal" and an "alternate" candidate for each vacancy.

A primary source of suggestions for candidates, at least for the scientific vacancies, is the staff of the institute. The staff is obviously conversant with the scientific requirements for council membership and the qualifications of suitable individuals. Other sources are the Congress, special interest groups, other DHHS agencies, the public, and current and past council members. The formal slate of nominations (ideally 25 percent of the membership of a council graduates each year) received from the NIH for each council is reviewed by the staff of the secretary. Decisions are finalized, factoring in political considerations, especially for lay representatives, and letters of invitations sent by the secretary to nominees.

TABLE 10.1. Distribution of M.D. and M.D./Ph.D. Council Members

Fiscal Year	Advisory Councils	Institute Review Committees	Study Sections
1979	56.4%	52.7%	42.3%
1985	62.0	53.5	35.4
1989	49.7	43.8	28.4

Membership of Advisory Councils

NIH Advisory Committees, a book published annually, contains rosters of all NIH advisory groups, including councils. Copies can be obtained from:

NIH Committee Management Office
Building 1, Room B1–56
Bethesda, MD 20892
(301) 496–2123

Some Characteristics of Council Members

Some of the principal findings from data compiled by DRG (DRG Peer Review Trends) covering the period from 1979–89, were:

- In FY 1989, there were 281 council members with scientific expertise. The distribution was 152 or 54.1 percent M.D.; 24 or 8.5 percent M.D./Ph.D.; 92 or 32.7 percent Ph.D.; and 13 or 4.7 percent other. Forty-five or 16 percent were women.
- The distribution of M.D. and M.D./Ph.D. members on various peer review groups is included in Table 10.1.
- Distribution of members by employing organizations is shown in Table 10.2.

TABLE 10.2. Distribution of Members by Employing Organization for FY 1989

	Advisory Councils	Institute Review Committees	Study Sections
Medical schools	38.3%	57.6%	56.3%
Other health professions schools	6.8	10.0	7.0
Other higher education	13.9	16.0	21.9
Independent hospitals	6.3	4.7	5.4
Nonprofit research organizations	12.0	8.9	8.4
Profit organizations	3.0	1.5	1.0
Other	19.7	1.3	0.0

The average age of council members in FY 1989 was 52.8 years. This is 5–7 years older than institute review committee members and 8 years older than study section members.

RULES THAT GOVERN THE FUNCTIONING
OF ADVISORY COUNCILS

The Public Health Service Act and NIH policy both set forth fundamental operating procedures for advisory councils. Other nonmandatory procedures are developed by an institute, usually in consultation with its council. A summary of both categories of council activities follows.

1. Review of applications for grants and cooperative agreements: The Public Health Service Act states that the "Directors of the national research institutes may award grants and cooperative agreements for research, training, and demonstration only if those awards have been recommended (a) after scientific/technical peer review, and (b) by the cognizant national advisory council when the annual direct cost of the award exceeds $50,000."

NIH strictly adheres to this requirement. Former minor loopholes in the process have been closed. For example, a council used to be able to accept either majority or minority recommendations in cases of split votes. However, at present, if a council does not agree with a scientific review group recommendation, it must return it for further review. Awards will not be made unless there is a favorable recommendation by both the review group and the council. In practice, there is excellent agreement in the recommendations at both review levels.

2. Program reviews: NIH policy requires that the director of each institute develop a procedure for periodically reviewing with its council the objectives, priorities, and accomplishments of each of its constituent programs, including intramural research. The frequency and details of such a plan must be approved by the Director, NIH. Program review presentations and discussions are conducted during the open or public portion of council meetings. The purpose of such reviews is to:

- Assure appropriate use of grant, cooperative agreement, and contract funds
- Provide information on program management
- Assure institute responsiveness to public needs
- Encourage new high-priority initiatives
- Assist the institute in establishing objectives and priorities, identifying resource requirements, and improving program management

3. Council operating guidelines: NIH policy requires institutes to develop, with their councils, mutually acceptable, formal guidelines permitting adjustments and modifications in awards by staff. This could be in time, amount, or other conditions of grants and applications previously recommended. Such guidelines are submitted to the Director, NIH, for approval and discussed at the first council meeting each fiscal year.

Examples of staff decisions not requiring prior council approval but presented after the fact for informational purposes follow:

- Requests by a grantee institution for a change in PI
- Requests by a PI to transfer a grant from one institution to another
- Award of administrative supplements for a variety of reasons, such as to cover institutional salary increases for personnel paid with grant funds; increases in institutional rates for animal care and maintenance; increases in hospital per diem costs
- Approval of extensions of grant periods for up to one year to insure orderly termination of the project. Extensions can be without funds or with prorated funds at a level no greater than the final year's support.

4. RFPs, RFAs, and PAs: The concept for an RFP must be approved by an advisory council or program advisory committee. Awarding units are required to consult with their council or a program advisory committee prior to issuing an RFA. For issuance of PAs, involvement of advisers is not required but encouraged.

NATIONAL ADVISORY COUNCIL MEETINGS

The law specifies that councils meet three times a year; for the NCI and NHLBI it is four times a year.

Meetings of councils are announced in the *Federal Register*. They are held on the NIH campus in Bethesda and can be up to three days in duration. A significant portion of each meeting is open to the public and is usually most informative. Agenda items include a report of the institute director updating happenings on the NIH scene and legislative and budgetary developments; program reviews; and discussion of new program initiatives. Meetings are closed for discussion of recommendations on grant and cooperative agreement applications.

Prior to each council meeting, members are sent summary statements of all applications to be considered at the meeting. Additionally, members are sent background and informational material on issues and agenda items to be brought up for discussion.

Discussion of grant applications can be considered by the council as a whole or in subcommittee sessions organized by major program areas. These groups meet either immediately before or during council meetings. Following these sessions, reports are presented to the full council for concurrence.

Review Procedures

Only certain types of applications are considered individually by the council. The vast majority have no obvious problems and the recommendations of scientific review groups are accepted without discussion. Examples of applications considered individually or as a group follow:

1. Applications are required to be brought to the attention of council if:
   - There are concerns raised by scientific review groups about animal welfare.
   - There are concerns raised by scientific review groups about research involving human subjects and potential biohazards.
   - The application is from a foreign institution and is considered for funding.
2. Other applications most often brought up for special discussion include:
   - Applications council members identify for discussion
   - Nonunanimous recommendations where there are both majority and minority opinions
   - Staff concerns with the scientific merit review
   - Applications with large recommended budgets, e.g., program projects and centers
   - Applications whose objectives are of special program interest or conversely of limited interest
3. MERIT Awards: Investigators do not apply for MERIT Awards. Staff makes recommendations for initial awards based on a minimum of the following published criteria; additional ones have been developed by individual institutes in consultation with councils:
   - The candidate must be PI on a competing R01 (new or renewal) that has been approved for five years with a percentile ranking better than 20 percent.
   - The candidate must have an impressive record of scientific achievement as the leader of one or more investigator-initiated research projects.
   - The candidate must be working actively in a research area that is of special importance or promise.

   Awardees are eligible for an extension of up to five years based on an abbreviated application which need only undergo review by staff and council.
4. Rebuttal letters: Rebuttal materials are made available to council regarding applications it is considering. Councils are asked to deal with review problems identified by staff and requests for restoration of reductions in time and amounts recommended by scientific review groups.
5. Responses to RFAs: Applications, along with review recommendations, are usually presented to council as a package for discussion and consideration of staff recommendations.

Recommendation Options

En bloc action: For all applications where a council agrees with scientific review group recommendations with no need for individual discussions, there is a motion for en bloc action. This encompasses approximately 98 percent of the applications on the council agenda.

Nonagreement with scientific merit recommendations: In such cases, there is a vote to return the application for rereview by the same study section, another study section, or for a project site visit.

Discussion of individual or groups of applications: Where indicated, votes are taken on motions based on staff or council recommendations, which may differ from those of the review group.

Deferrals: A council can defer an application for more information. Applications deferred by scientific review groups are not considered by a council until the initial review is complete.

Mail ballots: There are times when individual or groups of applications require council action between meetings. In such special cases, the staff can obtain a council vote by mail.

Priority Scores

Councils may not change the numerical priority scores assigned by scientific review groups. However, for certain types of council recommendations, alphabetic codes are used (see below) and included when a special council summary statement is prepared (see Chapter 11).

CON Concurrence with a numerical priority score

HPP High program priority—Recommended for funding out of numerical priority score/percentile order

LPP Low program priority—Essentially not recommended for funding no matter what the numerical priority score or percentile ranking.

OTH Other—Approval by council of an application that did not receive review by a scientific review group or some other unusual action. An example might be approval of an extension of a MERIT Award.

Between meetings, council members continue to be involved with institute business related to preparation of reports, subcommittee activities, or providing advice to staff when consulted.

GENERAL COMMENTS

Agendas of council meetings, meeting dates, well-documented minutes of meetings, council annual reports, and other council-related information can be obtained by contacting the executive secretary of the council (see list below). Attendance at council meetings can be very enlightening; if you are in the vicinity and the agenda includes items of interest, plan to attend. This can serve the dual purpose of information gathering and becoming better acquainted with staff.

Although DRG does not fund grants and contracts and has no legislatively mandated council, it does have an advisory committee, composed of distinguished

Executive Secretaries of National Advisory Councils

ICD	Address	Telephone
FIC	Building 31, Room B2C08	(301) 496–1491
NCI	Building 31, Room 10A03	(301) 496–5147
NCHGR	Building 38A, Room 605	(301) 496–0844
NCNR	Building 31, Room 5B10	(301) 496–0472
NCRR	Westwood Bldg., Room 10A03	(301) 496–6595
NEI	Building 31, Room 6A04	(301) 496–9110
NHLBI	Westwood Bldg., Room 7A17	(301) 496–7416
NIA	Gateway Building, Room 2C218	(301) 496–9322
NIAID	Solar Bldg., room 4C07	(301) 496–7291
NIAMS	Building 31, Room 4C32	(301) 496–0802
NICHD	Executive Plaza North, Room 520	(301) 496–1485
NIDCD	Executive Plaza South, Room 400	(301) 496–8693
NIDR	Westwood Building, Room 503	(301) 496–7723
NIDDK	Westwood Bldg., Room 657	(301) 496–7277
NIEHS	Building 3, Room 301A, P.O. Box 12233 Research Triangle Park, NC 27709	(919) 629–7723
NIGMS	Westwood Bldg., Room 938	(301) 496–7061
NINDS	Federal Bldg., Room 1016A	(301) 496–9248
NLM	Building 38, Room 2E17B	(301) 496–6221
DRG	Westwood Bldg., Room 449	(301) 496–7441

representatives of the scientific community, which meets twice annually. Their charge "is to provide technical and scientific advice to the Director, NIH, and the Director of the Division in two broad areas: first, review procedures and policies for the evaluation of grant applications for scientific and technical merit; and second, the development and management of modern information systems relevant to the support of biomedical and behavioral research and research training." This is a new committee, which held its first meeting in December 1989. The executive secretary can be contacted for more information (see accompanying chart).

National advisory councils are indispensable to the healthy functioning of the extramural programs. Aside from performing all the required council functions, and those that are not so obvious, their mere presence provides a tremendous incentive for staff to maintain high standards of performance. The staff expends a great deal of time and effort in preparing for council meetings. There must be a thorough familiarity with the applications to be considered along with the review group recommendations. All staff recommendations must be written up and distributed to members. A written record of council decisions must be prepared. Councils serve admirably to keep the staff on its toes and accountable for its actions.

11

Program Management

One of the most striking changes in the extramural programs began in the early 1970s. A high-level staff committee chaired by Dr. Theodore Cooper, then Director of the NHLBI, completed its study of the organization and management of the extramural programs. The resulting recommendations were implemented and the structure of the extramural programs was totally revamped. In the context of this chapter, the most relevant recommendations of the Cooper Committee were: (1) The extramural programs in each institute should be organized according to scientific program areas, and (2) the grant and contract mechanisms should be combined under single management within a program area.

Before these changes, institute programs, by and large, were organized by mechanism, e.g., research grants, training grants, program projects, centers, or contracts. This arrangement did not allow for adequate emphasis and coordination of the scientific content of the programs. An additional stimulus for change was the severe criticism from the scientific community about the peer review and management of contract proposals and programs. Thus, the findings of the Cooper Committee brought about a drastic realignment of staff activities and responsibilities and resulted in the current extramural organizational structure. Administrators with scientific backgrounds (Ph.D., M.D., or both), generically referred to as program staff, are in charge of the various program areas. To assist the program staff are grants management specialists who are conversant with grant policies and budget matters and contract specialists with analogous expertise in the contract realm. An 1989 NIH publication, *Orientation Handbook for Members of Scientific Review Groups*, summarizes the responsibilities of these NIH staff members as follows:

PROGRAM STAFF

- Develops program initiatives, such as RFAs
- Provides guidance and assistance to applicants
- Attends scientific review group (SRG) meetings to interpret program policy and provide other program information

- Provides SRG summary statements to applicants
- Presents SRG recommendations to council
- Makes award decisions
- Participates in identifying prospective SRG and council nominees
- Evaluates accomplishments of scientific programs
- Monitors research progress during award periods

GRANTS AND CONTRACTS MANAGEMENT STAFF

- Provides business management guidance to applicants and reviewers
- Attends SRG meetings
- Attends council meetings
- Participates with program staff in budget negotiations prior to and following awards
- Maintains official grant and contract files
- Assists in development of program policy
- Brings fiscal and policy expertise to the management of grant and contract programs
- Provides fiscal management expertise

The above summary only highlights the important role these staff members play in the extramural review and award process. Get to know the staff, particularly in the areas of science and administration over which they have specific jurisdiction (see listing at the end of the chapter). For the most part, you will find the staff knowledgeable, cooperative, and willing to offer advice. They will not be able to deliver a grant award, but they should be able to remove some of the anxiety from the grant-seeking process. To provide more detail about staff activities and to emphasize how they can assist applicants and awardees, tracking an application through the different stages of the grant process should prove helpful.

BEFORE SUBMITTING AN APPLICATION

Program staff can provide information on a number of matters, such as:

An institute's program interests: The staff can describe and elaborate on an institute's broad and special research interests, informative brochures, and staff contacts. If you are working in a basic science discipline, keep in mind that institutes usually like to attract new disciplines or scientific approaches. Most are quite liberal in their interpretation of program acceptability. However, make sure any application submitted makes a reasonable attempt to relate research objectives to program interests.

An institute's mechanisms of support: Not all institutes sponsor all mechanisms. Detailed descriptions of individual NIH mechanisms are available. Chapter 4 and Appendixes 2 and 3 provide only topical information. You will undoubtedly need more detail about availability, suitability, criteria, etc., and any special requirements indigenous to a particular institute. Also, there are always new mechanisms being developed and, in some cases, older ones being phased out.

Comments on draft proposals: Program staff should be willing to review draft proposals. They will not offer opinions on the quality of the science but can advise on issues such as relevance to the institute's programs; changes to include in an amended application; omissions or deviations from the instructions for filling out the application; adequacy of budget justifications and explanations of interrelation of the project(s) with other support; and grant policy issues. In the case of program projects or similar type center applications, there are a number of other essential ingredients that may benefit from staff feedback, e.g., presence of a focused central theme and the relationship of individual projects to it; the evidence for proper coordination and management of the program; and presence of sufficient expertise and research to support the program.

As a general rule, it is unwise to submit large, unsolicited proposals without some form of staff contact. Aside from program projects and centers, another example is a multisite clinical trial. The staff will appreciate learning about such plans and welcome the opportunity to comment before a formal application submission, if the proposal is unsolicited and not in response to an RFA.

Application procedures: If the program staff has been discussing an application with you, they may be able to help with the referral process, as explained in Chapter 6. Additionally, they can answer questions about a multitude of application review and award procedures that may cause you concern.

INITIAL REVIEW

After an application is submitted, it has to be assigned, processed, duplicated, and distributed. Therefore, many weeks elapse before it finds its way to the desks of the program administrator and grants management specialist responsible for following it through the system. The vast majority of applications fit an institute's program guidelines either because they have been previously screened, e.g., they are amendments, renewals, and supplements, or the assignment is straightforward. If there is a problem with an institute assignment, program staff will notify the DRG Referral Office. The assignment to a scientific review group is also checked not only for fit but also for potential problems. Examples are conflict of interest situations, repeated assignment of resubmissions to the same study section, and incompatibility with council recommendations. These matters are usually discussed informally with the SRA.

Aside from assignment checks, the applications are scrutinized in preparation for the staff's attendance at the review group meeting. Items examined are current level of support for supplements and renewals, budget justifications, questions of overlap with other support, and past review and award history. If there are concerns, the program administrator will discuss these with the SRA either before or privately during the meeting. Program administrators and grants management personnel are observers at review group meetings, do not get involved in discussions unless invited to do so, but must be prepared to answer questions. However, they listen to the discussions and take notes. The notes can serve as a supplemental source of information to the summary statement if they contain anything new and different, and if the subject of such additional information is raised by the applicant or staff. As an aside, do not be surprised if the program administrator in charge of your application did not attend the review meeting. Ideally, program administrators should be present at the discussion of all applications assigned to them. However, with the large number of review meetings being held during a relatively short time period, schedule conflicts may preclude this type of coverage by the same staff member and others are asked to help out.

Immediately following the meeting, the program staff will obviously be aware of the recommendations but not the priority scores or percentile ratings. Approximately ten weeks are required before summary statements are prepared and released. It is unfair to expect the program administrator to engage in a discussion of the scientific review until the summary statement is available. Before release, summary statements are reviewed by program and grants management staff for inaccuracies, inconsistencies, inappropriate statements, and policy or other problems. If changes are indicated, the SRA is notified. After release, it is quite common for investigators to call program administrators to discuss the content of summary statements. This is a good opportunity for PIs to obtain an additional perspective of the review, information about funding status, advice on whether and how to proceed with a resubmission, and information about rebuttal and appeal procedures.

COUNCIL REVIEW

Program and grants management staff expend considerable time and effort preparing for council meetings. Summary statements are reviewed to identify those in need of council attention. Staff meetings are held to discuss application recommendations, rebuttal materials, and proposed staff recommendations to be presented to the council. The types of applications that are discussed by the council are listed in Chapter 10. Several issues warrant additional mention here.

Rebuttal Letters

Rebuttal letters become the responsibility of the program administrator once the DRG Study Section or ICD committee review has been completed. Assuming you are unhappy with some aspect of the review, should you submit a letter? Before doing so, discuss the matter with the program administrator who will be receiving the letter and dealing with the problem. In the case of complaints about the review process, the program administrator will try to determine if the review was carried out in a satisfactory manner by discussion with the SRA, other staff, and, if necessary, individual reviewers. If there are no apparent problems with the review, the applicant will likely be advised to resubmit. If the review is flawed and there is agreement between program administrator and SRA, the staff has the authority to defer the application for further review without taking it to the council. If there is no agreement, the program administrator will arrange to have the rebuttal material reviewed by the council. Other common types of rebuttal letters are those requesting restoration of reductions in time and amount. In cases of restorations of time, the case is referred to the council. In cases of restoration of funds, some institutes allow the staff to handle the matter without advice from the Council. Do not overlook the key role program administrators play in the rebuttal procedure! They have the option of obtaining additional scientific opinions, if necessary; arranging for council review, if indicated; and preparing staff recommendations for council consideration, if advisable (see Chapter 12 for more detailed information).

MERIT Awards

Applicants do not apply for the award but are nominated by program administrators from the pool of competing applications. Based on published criteria and refinements developed by individual institutes, a staff recommendation is prepared for the initial five-year award. The council must approve each application nominated for a MERIT Award.

Extensions of three to five years are permitted with an abbreviated application using the PHS 398 kit. All that is required for the Research Plan portion of the application is a progress report, prepared according to the PHS 398 instructions, and a one-page abstract of the research plan for the extension period. No review by a scientific review group is required. Instead, program and grants management staff review the application, the original application and summary statement, interim progress reports, resulting publications, and prepare a recommendation to include budget levels. The council must review and approve extensions.

Responses to RFAs

Program administrators usually will prepare a document for the council that summarizes the scientific objectives of the RFA, describes the review process used to evaluate applications, provides statistics related to the competition, recommends applications to be funded, offers an explanation of how the funded projects would achieve the goals of the RFA, and presents a budget plan for the initial and subsequent years of support.

Council Meetings

Staff activity heightens prior to each council meeting. Books of summary statements have to be compiled and mailed out in time to allow council members to read them. Computer lists of competing applications are generated in a variety of ways to assist council members and staff in locating summary statements and reviewing ratings and budget information. Written recommendations have to be prepared for applications requiring special council action. There is a host of other paperwork and details related to council meeting preparation which the staff has to accomplish.

After the council meeting, there is another surge of activity on the part of the program staff. A number of follow-up items must be looked after:

Preparation of council summary statements: These are prepared for those applications where the council has taken an action different from the recommendation of the scientific review group, e.g., deferral or restoration of time and amount or when a special council action is required, such as funding an application from a foreign institution. Such summary statements become part of the official grant file and thus are subject to release, upon request, under the provisions of the Privacy Act.

Preparation of routine letters to applicants: These fall into three categories, with modifications when necessary.

1. Notification to applicants of an intent to fund
2. Notification of an uncertain funding status
3. Notification of an unfundable application

Notifications of "not for further consideration" and "too low a percentile (lower one-third) to be further considered" are sent out prior to council meetings.

Preparation of special letters to applicants: These relate to the following situations:

- Responses to rebuttal letters
- Deferral of funding decisions because of questions of overlap, ethical issues, women and minority representation in study populations, and problems with other grant policy issues
- Extensions without funds for not-to-be funded renewal applications
- Extensions with funds, under certain circumstances, for not-to-be funded renewal applications
- Human subject issues

- Animal welfare issues
- Council deferral recommendations for rereview or for more information. Also, in cases of rereviews, memos are required notifying SRAs of scientific review groups of the reasons for another review.
- Notification to a foreign institution of an intent to fund an application. Such letters are sent after State Department clearance is obtained.
- Other miscellaneous letters as required.

In essence, at least one letter is needed for each application reviewed.

At this point, an application has worked its way through the peer review system and decisions on funding eligibility have been made. However, the duties of the program administrator are by no means over.

OTHER ACTIVITIES OF A PROGRAM ADMINISTRATOR

Award Issues

There are three grant cycles per fiscal year. Therefore, an institute's grant budget has to be portioned out properly to ensure that awards can be made after each council meeting, e.g., 30 percent for the first council meeting of the fiscal year (October), 30 percent for the second meeting (February), and 40 percent for the last meeting (May). In addition, the funds set aside for each council meeting have to be distributed to the major program areas within an institute. In the case of the NHLBI, the distribution is stipulated by law; no less than 15 percent for the lung programs and no less than 15 percent for the blood programs. This may make it difficult to maintain a uniform institute payline because one program may be able to fund more applications with its budget allotment than another. Each institute develops its own method of establishing program and institute paylines.

In most cases, paylines are not absolute. Everyone wants to fund the highest quality research. Therefore, the usual practice is to start funding applications with the highest percentile ratings and to work downward toward the payline. Institutes vary in the latitude delegated to staff in making funding decisions, particularly for applications near the payline, where percentile differences are not too significant. For example, an institute may give preference near the payline to certain types of applications such as those from investigators with no other research support or renewals or for research of special interest. Depending on the institute, program administrators usually have authority to make certain funding decisions. In FY 1990, over 11.5 percent of competing research project grant applications were paid out of order either by staff or council recommendation. This percentage for the individual ICDs ranged between 3.3 percent and 30 percent and should indicate that other factors aside from merit can enter into funding decisions.

TABLE 11.1. FY 1990 Institute Percentile Paylines for RPGs

Institute	Success Rate	Theoretical Percentile Payline*
NIH	24.0	19.9
NIA	21.4	24.0
NIAID	27.2	22.0
NIAMS	20.0	16.3
NCI	23.5	20.0
NICHD	19.3	15.9
NIDCD	36.9	29.5
NIDR	20.9	18.5
NIDDK	23.0	18.3
NIEHS	28.3	30.5
NEI	37.5	33.8
NIGMS	22.0	16.1
NHLBI	24.9	20.1
NINDS	24.2	20.2
NCNR	16.4	18.7
NCHGR	23.3	23.3
NCRR	21.6	Insufficient data

*Does not include SBIRs (R43 and R44).

Source: Extramural Trends, FY 1981-1990.

As a point of interest, data on the theoretical institute percentile paylines are available for FY 1990 and are presented in Table 11.1.

Also, program administrators are involved in identifying applications eligible for James A. Shannon Awards. Applicants do not apply for a Shannon Award. R01 and R29 applications are peer reviewed in the usual manner. Those applications falling beyond the funding payline, but where the perceived quality is not significantly different from those funded, will be considered. Nominations are submitted by ICD staff through their institute directors to OD/NIH. A committee of senior NIH officials makes recommendations to the NIH director, who will use discretionary funds and transfer authority to make these awards. Awards provide up to $100,000 in total costs ($80,000 direct costs and $20,000 indirect costs) for a twenty-four-month period (see Appendix 2).

After funding decisions are made, the program and grants management staff work in tandem to take care of the details associated with making an award. If there are questions of overlap with existing support, the facts will be gathered from other institutes or agencies, e.g., NSF, and the applicant institution. The program administrator has the option of obtaining assistance from scientific consultants, if necessary, to arrive at a negotiated budget. If there are questions about the use of human subjects or animals, these must be satisfactorily resolved in order to make an award. Budgets are carefully checked and adjusted to recommended or negotiated levels and individual items such as consortium arrangements, subcontracts, leasing agreements, and patients costs are examined. When the requisite preparatory work is complete, the Notice of Grant Award is issued.

Postaward Issues

Several matters arise during award periods that require administrative decisions other than those delegated to grantee institutions. For example, requests from a PI who is moving to a new institution and wishes to take along a grant fall into this category. A relinquishing statement from the current institution and an application from the new institution assuring the availability of adequate facilities and personnel to continue the project are required. The program administrator has the option of approving the request, denying it, or seeking advice from scientific consultants. Other examples are: requests from a PI to significantly alter the research objectives of a project; requests from a grantee institution to name a new PI, either temporarily (more than ninety days) or permanently; or requests for changes in other personnel essential to the success of the project. Before formal requests are filed, it may prove helpful to discuss the situation with the program administrator.

Noncompeting Applications

Grantee institutions must submit, annually, a noncompeting application (PHS 2590) to continue to receive funding throughout the project period of an award. Evaluation of progress is the responsibility of the program and grants management staff. The application is considered important by the staff in that it is used to identify significant scientific advances and research accomplishments that have occurred with an institute's grant support during a fiscal year. These are reported to Congress, the public, special interest groups, and other government agencies in a variety of ways.

Dr. Stephen Gordon (Program Administrator, NIAMS) and Ms. Diane Watson (Grants Management Officer, NIAMS) in their paper (1990), "Use and Importance of the NIH Noncompeting Continuation Application," present the need for a thoughtfully prepared application:

> The following guidelines for preparing the application are suggested to assist program staff glean the most significant findings, including the effect the investigator's research has on its field.
>
> The Progress Report Summary identifies the scientific accomplishments of the grant. Generally, the writing style should be targeted to an informed lay reader (i.e., similar to that of *Scientific American*). Technical details should be sufficient for the

reader to understand the progress, but not to the extent necessary when publishing the research results. A clear and concise report is invaluable to NIH staff.

A separate significance section would be useful to program staff as they review the application. This could be one or two paragraphs, written in layman's terms, summarizing the key findings and their significance, and including both basic and applied research advances. Opportunities for further investigations made possible by these recent results should be identified. The effect these findings might have on medical intervention should be mentioned. If the results require further verification with additional statistics, this too should be indicated. It may also be helpful to comment on the relation of this project to overall progress in the field of research.

Even though approval is routine except in unusual circumstances, the time invested in reviewing the content of each noncompeting application in a program administrator's grant portfolio is considerable. The progress report and plans for the future are examined, as well as budgetary details and assurances of compliance with PHS policy, e.g., research protocols involving human subjects.

RFA Programs

Many RFAs require that grantees meet periodically to exchange information and report on progress. The program administrator overseeing the RFA is responsible for the planning and conduct of such meetings. Also, after the RFA grant period is over, some programs require the program administrator to prepare a report evaluating the success of the initiative.

Centers

The management of center programs varies among institutes because of the different objectives and types of center programs. Some program managers may supplement information in annual progress reports, submitted with noncompeting applications, by conducting periodic site visits during the grant period. Others may convene meetings of center participants to discuss scientific findings and to encourage collaboration. Whatever the approach used by an institute, program administrators in charge of center programs are involved in all the details related to their monitoring together with their grants management colleagues.

New Initiatives

Ideas generated from workshops, conferences, or program advisory committees must go through a series of prioritization and approval steps and then be developed into RFAs and RFPs. Program administrators are involved in each step of the planning and implementation for these institute-initiated projects.

Contacts for Major ICD Program Areas

ICD and Program Area	Address	Telephone
NIA		
Biology of Aging Program	Gateway Building, Room 2C231	(301) 496–4996
Molecular and Cellular Biology Program	Gateway Building, Room 2C231	(301) 496–6402
Geriatrics Program	Gateway Building, Room 3E327	(301) 496–6761
Behavioral and Social Research Program	Gateway Building, Room 2C234	(301) 496–3136
Neuroscience and Neuropsychology of Aging Program	Gateway Building, Room 3C307	(301) 496–9350
NIAID		
Allergy, Immunology, and Transplantation	Solar Building, Room 4A16	(301) 496–1886
Asthma and Allergy	Solar Bldg., Room 4A23	(301) 496–8973
Basic Immunology	Solar Bldg., Room 4A22	(301) 496–7551
Genetics and Transplantation	Solar Bldg., Room 4A14	(301) 496–5598
Clinical Immunology	Solar Bldg., Room 4A19	(301) 496–7104
Microbiology and Infectious Diseases	Solar Building, Room 3A18	(301) 496–1884
Clinical and Regulatory Affairs	Solar Building, Room 3A01	(301) 496–2126
Antiviral Research	Solar Bldg., Room 3A22	(301) 496–7051
Enteric Diseases	Solar Bldg., Room 3A05	(301) 496–7051
Respiratory Diseases	Solar Bldg., Room 3A08	(301) 496–7051
Sexually Transmitted Diseases	Solar Bldg., Room 3A20	(301) 402–0443
Epidemiology and Biometry	Solar Bldg., Room 3A24	(301) 496–7065
Virology	Solar Bldg., Room 3A16	(301) 496–7453
Parasitology and Tropical Diseases	Solar Bldg., Room 3A02	(301) 496–2544
Bacteriology and Mycology	Solar Bldg., Room 3A04	(301) 496–8285
Acquired Immunodeficiency Syndrome (AIDS)	Solar Bldg., Room 2A18	(301) 496–0545
Community Clinical Research	Solar Bldg., Room 2C26	(301) 496–0701
Epidemiology	Solar Bldg., Room 2A42	(301) 496–6177
Biostatistics Research	Solar Bldg., Room 2B27	(301) 496–0694
Treatment Research	Solar Bldg., Room 2C19	(301) 496–8210
Clinical Trials Resources	Solar Bldg., Room 2A04	(301) 496–8214
Basic Research and Development	Solar Bldg., Room 2C07	(301) 496–0638
Vaccine Research and Development	Solar Bldg., Room 2B01	(301) 496–8200
Pathogenesis	Solar Bldg., Room 2B33	(301) 496–8378
Developmental Therapeutics	Solar Bldg., Room 2C11	(301) 496–8199
Resources and Centers	Solar Bldg., Room 2B31	(301) 496–0755
NIAMS		
Rheumatic Diseases	Westwood Bldg., Room 405B	(301) 496–7326
Muscle Biology	Westwood Bldg., Room 403B	(301) 496–7495
Musculoskeletal Diseases	Westwood Bldg., Room 407A	(301) 496–7326
Bone Diseases	Westwood Bldg., Room 403D	(301) 496–7495
Skin Diseases	Westwood Bldg., Room 405A	(301) 496–7326
Centers Program	Westwood Bldg., Room 403C	(301) 496–7495

(continued)

Contacts for Major ICD Program Areas (*Continued*)

ICD and Program Area	Address	Telephone
NCI		
Cancer Diagnosis	Executive Plaza South, Room 638	(301) 496–1591
Cancer Biology	Executive Plaza South, Room 630	(301) 496–7028
Cancer Immunology	Executive Plaza South, Room 634	(301) 496–7815
Centers, Training and Resources	Executive Plaza North, Room 308	(301) 496–8531
Biological Carcinogenesis	Executive Plaza North, Room 540	(301) 496–9740
Chemical and Physical Carcinogenesis	Executive Plaza North, Room 700N	(301) 496–5471
Epidemiology and Biostatistics	Executive Plaza North, Room 543	(301) 496–1611
Radiation Research	Executive Plaza North, Room 800	(301) 496–6111
Developmental Therapeutics	Executive Plaza North, Room 843	(301) 496–8720
Cancer Therapy Evaluation	Executive Plaza North, Room 742F	(301) 496–6138
Cancer Prevention Research	Executive Plaza North, Room 200	(301) 496–8567
Cancer Control Science Program	Executive Plaza North, Room 243B	(301) 496–8594
Early Detection and Community Oncology	Executive Plaza North, Room 300H	(301) 496–8541
Surveillance Program	Executive Plaza North, Room 343M	(301) 496–8506
NICHD		
Population Research	Executive Plaza North, Room 604	(301) 496–1101
Contraceptive Development	Executive Plaza North, Room 600	(301) 496–1661
Demographics and Behavioral Sciences	Executive Plaza North, Room 611	(301) 496–1174
Reproductive Sciences	Executive Plaza North, Room 603	(301) 496–6515
Contraceptive and Reproductive Evaluation	Executive Plaza North, Room 607	(301) 496–4924
Research for Mothers and Children	Executive Plaza North, Room 643	(301) 496–5097
Genetics and Teratology	Executive Plaza North, Room 643	(301) 496–5541
Mental Retardation and Developmental Disabilities	Executive Plaza North, Room 631	(301) 496–1383
Human Learning and Behavior	Executive Plaza North, Room 633	(301) 496–6591
Endocrinology, Nutrition, and Growth	Executive Plaza North, Room 637	(301) 496–5593
Pregnancy and Perinatology	Executive Plaza North, Room 643	(301) 496–5575
Pediatric, Adolescent and Maternal AIDS	Executive Plaza South, Room 450 West	(301) 496–7339
NIDCD		
Hearing Program	Executive Plaza South, Room 400	(301) 496–5061
Voice, Speech, and Language Program	Executive Plaza South, Room 400	(301) 496–5061
Chemical Senses Program	Executive Plaza South, Room 400	(301) 496–5061
Vestibular Program	Executive Plaza South, Room 400	(301) 496–5061
NIDR		
Periodontal Diseases	Westwood Bldg., Room 507	(301) 496–778
Caries, Nutrition and Flouride	Westwood Bldg., Room 505	(301) 496–788
Craniofacial Development and Disorders	Westwood Bldg., Room 506	(301) 496–780
Biomaterials, Pulp Biology and Implants	Westwood Bldg., Room 505	(301) 496–788
Oral Soft Tissue Diseases and AIDS	Westwood Bldg., Room 507	(301) 496–778

(*continued*)

Contacts for Major ICD Program Areas (*Continued*)

ICD and Program Area	Address	Telephone
Salivary Glands and Oral Biology	Westwood Bldg., Room 505	(301) 496–7884
Behavior, Pain, Oral Motor and Oral Sensory and Epidemiology	Westwood Bldg., Room 506	(301) 496–7807
NIDDK		
Diabetes Research	Westwood Bldg., Room 622	(301) 496–7731
Diabetes Centers Program	Westwood Bldg., Room 626	(301) 496–7418
Endocrinology Research	Westwood Bldg., Room 621	(301) 496–7504
Cystic Fibrosis	Westwood Bldg., Room 625	(301) 496–4980
Metabolic Diseases	Westwood Bldg., Room 625	(301) 496–7997
Liver and Biliary Diseases	Westwood Bldg., Room 3A17	(301) 496–7858
Pancreas Program	Westwood Bldg., Room 3A18A	(301) 496–7121
GI Digestion	Westwood Bldg., Room 3A18A	(301) 496–7121
GI Immunology	Westwood Bldg., Room 3A18A	(301) 496–7121
GI Neuroendocrinology	Westwood Bldg., Room 3A16	(301) 496–7821
GI Mobility	Westwood Bldg., Room 3A16	(301) 496–7821
Digestive Diseases Centers Program	Westwood Bldg., Room 3A15	(301) 496–9717
Nutrition Program	Westwood Bldg., Room 3A18	(301) 496–7823
Renal Physiology and Cell Biology	Westwood Bldg., Room 3A04A	(301) 496–7459
Urology	Westwood Bldg., Room 3A05B	(301) 496–8248
Chronic Renal Disease	Westwood Bldg., Room 3A07A	(301) 496–8218
HIV Program	Westwood Bldg., Room 3A05A	(301) 496–8218
End State Renal Disease	Westwood Bldg., Room 3A11A	(301) 496–7571
Hematology	Westwood Bldg., Room 3A05C	(301) 496–7458
NIEHS		
Biometry and Risk Assessment	Building 3, Room 305A P.O. Box 12233 Research Triangle Park, NC 27709	(919) 629–7634
Toxicology Research and Testing	Building 3, Room 305A P.O. Box 12233 Research Triangle Park, NC 27709	(919) 629–7634
Biological Responses to Environmental Agents	Building 3, Room 305A P.O. Box 12233 Research Triangle Park, NC 27709	(919) 629–7634
NEI		
Retinal and Choroidal Diseases	Building 31, Room 6A48	(301) 496–5884
Corneal Diseases	Building 31, Room 6A48	(301) 496–5884
Cataract	Building 31, Room 6A48	(301) 496–5884
Glaucoma	Building 31, Room 6A48	(301) 496–5884
Strabismus, Amblyopia, and Visual Processing	Building 31, Room 6A47	(301) 496–5301

(*continued*)

Contacts for Major ICD Program Areas (*Continued*)

ICD and Program Area	Address	Telephone
NIGMS		
Cellular and Molecular Basis of Disease	Westwood Bldg., Room 903	(301) 496–7021
Genetics Program	Westwood Bldg., Room 910	(301) 496–7175
Pharmacological Sciences	Westwood Bldg., Room 919	(301) 496–7707
Biophysics and Physiological Sciences	Westwood Bldg., Room 907	(301) 496–7463
Minority Access to Research (MARC)	Westwood Bldg., Room 950	(301) 496–7941
Minority Biomedical Research Support (MBRSP)	Westwood Bldg., Room 952	(301) 496–6745
NHLBI		
Heart and Vascular Diseases	Federal Bldg., Room 416A	(301) 496–2553
Cardiology	Federal Bldg., Room 320	(301) 496–5421
Cardiac Diseases	Federal Bldg., Room 3C06	(301) 496–1081
Cardiac Functions	Federal Bldg., Room 304C	(301) 496–1627
Devices and Technology	Federal Bldg., Room 312A	(301) 496–1586
Arteriosclerosis, Hypertension and Lipid Metabolism	Federal Bldg., Room 4C12A	(301) 496–1613
Behavioral Medicine	Federal Bldg., Room 216	(301) 496–9380
Clinical Trials	Federal Bldg., Room 5C01	(301) 496–4323
Prevention and Demonstration Research	Federal Bldg., Room 604	(301) 496–2465
Lung Diseases	Westwood Bldg., Room 6A16	(301) 496–7208
Cell and Developmental Biology	Westwood Bldg., Room 6A07	(301) 496–7171
Airways Diseases	Westwood Bldg., Room 6A15	(301) 496–7332
Interstitial Lung Diseases	Westwood Bldg., Room 6A09	(301) 496–7034
Prevention, Education and Research Training	Westwood Bldg., Room 640	(301) 496–7668
Blood Diseases and Resources	Federal Bldg., Room 516B	(301) 496–4868
Bone Marrow Transplantation	Federal Bldg., Room 5C04	(301) 496–8387
Cellular Hematology	Federal Bldg., Room 5A12	(301) 496–1537
Transfusion Medicine	Federal Bldg., Room 504	(301) 496–1537
Thrombosis and Hematosis	Federal Bldg., Room 516C	(301) 496–8966
Sickle Cell Disease	Federal Bldg., Room 504D	(301) 496–6931
NINDS		
Fundamental Neurosciences	Federal Bldg., Room 916	(301) 496–5745
Convulsive, Developmental, and Neuromuscular Disorders	Federal Bldg., Room 816B	(301) 496–6541
Epilepsy	Federal Bldg., Room 114	(301) 496–6691
Developmental Neurology	Federal Bldg., Room 8C10	(301) 496–6701
Demyelinating, Atrophic, and Dementing Disorders	Federal Bldg., Room 810A	(301) 496–5679
Stroke and Trauma	Federal Bldg., Room 8A08A	(301) 496–2581
NLM		
Biomedical Information	Building 38A, Room 5S522	(301) 496–4221
International Programs	Building 38A, Room 5N519	(301) 496–6131

(*continued*)

Contacts for Major ICD Program Areas (*Continued*)

ICD and Program Area	Address	Telephone
NCHGR		
Genetic Mapping	Building 38A, Room 612	(301) 496–7531
Physical Mapping	Building 38A, Room 612	(301) 496–7531
Sequencing	Building 38A, Room 612	(301) 496–7531
Ethical, Legal, and Social Issues	Building 38A, Room 617	(301) 402–0911
Genome Informatics	Building 38A, Room 612	(301) 496–7531
Technology Development	Building 38A, Room 614	(301) 496–7531
Research Centers	Building 38A, Room 610	(301) 496–7531
NCNR		
Acute and Chronic Illnesses	Building 31, Room 5B11	(301) 496–0523
Health Promotion and Disease Prevention	Building 31, Room 5B11	(301) 496–0523
Nursing Systems	Building 31, Room 5B11	(301) 496–0523
NCRR		
Animal Resources	Westwood Building, Room 857	(301) 496–5175
Biological Models and Material Resources	Westwood Bldg., Room 8A07	(301) 402–0630
Biomedical Research Support Program (BRSP)	Westwood Bldg., Room 10A11	(301) 496–6743
Biomedical Research Technology Program	Westwood Bldg., Room 8A15	(301) 496–5411
General Clinical Research Centers	Westwood Bldg., Room 10A03	(301) 496–6595
Research Centers in Minority Institutions	Westwood Bldg., Room 10A10	(301) 496–6341
Research Facilities Improvement Program	Westwood Bldg., Room 8A15	(301) 496–8482
FIC		
International AIDS Training Grants	Building 31, Room B2C39	(301) 496–1653
International Fellowships	Building 31, Room B2C39	(301) 496–1653
Foreign Currency Programs	Building 31, Room B2C39	(301) 496–6688

GENERAL COMMENTS

Attention has been focused on program administrators and grants management staff and the role they play in the extramural review and award process. We hope the information will provide some useful insights into the duties of the program staff and the timing of their activities. Be sure to consider taking advantage of the services and assistance the program staff can offer! The accompanying charts contain the addresses and telephone numbers for the major ICD programs and the grants management officers.

Grants Management Officers

ICD	Address	Telephone
FIC	Building 31, Room B2C39	(301) 496–1653
NCI	Executive Plaza South, Room 234	(301) 496–7753
NCHGR	Building 38A, Room 613	(301) 402–0733
NCNR	Building 31, Room 5B06	(301) 496–0237
NCRR	Westwood Bldg., Room 853	(301) 496–9840
NEI	Building 31, Room 6A48	(301) 496–5884
NHLBI	Westwood Bldg., Room 4A12B	(301) 496–7255
NIA	Gateway Building, Room 2N212	(301) 496–1472
NIAID	Solar Bldg., Room 4B21	(301) 496–7231
NIAMS	Westwood Bldg., Room 407A	(301) 496–7495
NICHD	Executive Plaza North, Room 501	(301) 496–5001
NIDCD	Executive Plaza South, Room 400	(301) 402–0909
NIDR	Westwood Bldg., Room 518	(301) 496–7437
NIDDK	Westwood Bldg., Room 653	(301) 496–7467
NIEHS	Building 2, Room 203B P.O. Box 12233 Research Triangle Park, NC 27709	(919) 629–7628
NIGMS	Westwood Bldg., Room 953	(301) 496–7746
NINDS	Federal Bldg., Room 1004A	(301) 496–9231
NLM	Building 38A, Room 5N509	(301) 496–4253

12

Decision Points and Communications and Appeals

While it is important for a PI to know what to do, and when and how to do it in applying for grant support, it is also valuable to know where the critical decision points are in the process. This will avoid time-consuming delays in the processing and review of applications.

DECISION POINTS

At the Applicant Institution

Because so much depends on the award of a grant, useful advice from experienced researchers and administrators should be sought. Where appropriate, the completed draft of the application should be discussed with knowledgeable *senior faculty members* of the department. There may be a departmental *publications committee* organized to approve the submission of applications as well as research papers for publication.

Some departments in some institutions have their own *business office* through which applications must pass before going to the institutional *Office of Grants and Contracts* or the *Office of Sponsored Research*. This latter office is usually involved to assure that all the rules and regulations are followed, provide the institutional official's signature, and set into motion the process of tracking applications through the various stages. They may also comment on the science of the proposed projects and provide valuable advice on the application content or the grants process. This office also should be contacted to complete Form PHS 6315, which deals with misconduct in science, and to provide the information required in the Checklist assuring a drug-free workplace. The institution's *business office* has the last word on the structure and content of the PI's requested budget.

If human subjects are involved in the proposed research, the *Institutional Review Board* must review and approve the protocols. If vertebrate animals are to be used, the *Institutional Animal Care and Use Committee* must approve the maintenance, care, and choice of species, in addition to the research protocols and the method of euthanasia for the animals. In either case, sufficient time must be allowed for these panels to complete their work so that the application can be submitted to meet the proper receipt date.

At the NIH

The first decisions made at the NIH are in the *Referral Office* of the Division of Research Grants. If the application arrives after the receipt date, the Referral Office determines whether it should be accepted. It then must be determined that it is complete administratively. A *DRG referral officer* will examine the application to see if it is health related and thus appropriate for support from the USPHS. It will also be determined whether it is a new application, a competing continuation, or a supplement or a revision of an earlier submission. Finally, decisions will be made as to the assignments to an ICD(s) for potential funding and to a review panel for scientific merit evaluation.

In the *Study Section Office*, the application is reviewed again to see if it is assigned appropriately and whether it is complete both administratively and scientifically. The *scientific review administrator* must decide if any conflict of interest situations exist and which of the members will be assigned in-depth review responsibilities. A decision will also be made regarding the need for opinions from outside experts or the need for ad hoc (special) reviewers to participate in the meeting.

In the *study section meeting*, the *reviewers* are expected to recommend that the application be given consideration, no further consideration, or deferral. If the decision is to defer, the panel members then must decide if the required additional information can be obtained by mail or by a project site visit and, if a site visit, what sort of expertise would be needed at the visit. Finally, if the application is to be given consideration, the panel members recommend a budget, a project period, and assign a priority rating.

The *funding component staff* either concurs with the study section recommendation or suggests to the advisory council some modification of the recommendation, such as restoration of deleted budget items or years of support. They may even recommend deferral for a site visit or that the application be rereviewed by the same or another study section.

The *advisory council* or *board* will either concur with the study section, the recommendation of the ICD program staff, or present a recommendation of its own. In addition, the council, on the basis of previous programmatic decisions, may also designate an application to be of high or low program priority. In the former case, the application usually will be funded and, in the latter case, will remain unfunded regardless of priority score or percentile rating.

The *ICD director* has the final decision on funding an application. If the decision is to fund, the *grants management staff* may either process funding as recommended or negotiate a budget with the applicant institution.

COMMUNICATIONS AND APPEALS

The grant peer review system has become large and complex, with a multitude of players, and every attempt is made to keep it fair and objective. In most cases, when a PI objects to a particular action, honest differences of opinion are at play. However, it is a human system and mistakes are made, and applicant investigators have the opportunity to dispute decisions and recommendations, present their points of view, and seek redress from real or perceived wrongs.

In the past, the system of appeals at NIH was informal. The PI wrote a letter to program or review staff rebutting the review, and program and review staff would collaborate on a response, sometimes with outside advice. For the most part, the matter usually resulted in submission of a revised proposal. Because honest differences of opinion have been at the heart of most disagreements, this approach was encouraged.

Changes came about in the late 1970s as a result of studies by an NIH staff Grants Peer Review Study Team, organized to look at all aspects of the NIH peer review system. Among its recommendations, adopted by the director of NIH, was the institution of a formal appeals system encompassing the entire process of the peer review of an application, from receipt and assignment through advisory council review. This resulted in a system of communications (rebuttals) and appeals, the purpose of which is to ensure a thorough examination of the applicant's concerns, a response matching the appeal in kind, and assurance that these concerns are handled promptly and efficiently. In this new system, the following areas became appealable:

- The acceptance of an application by NIH
- Assignment to a funding component or to a review panel
- The composition of the review committee or a project site visit team where expertise, conflict of interest, or possible bias might be of concern
- The study section recommendations
- The advisory council recommendations
- The ICD staff actions

On the other hand, the appeals process is not intended to:

- Bypass the peer review process
- Resolve purely scientific disputes (honest differences of scientific opinion) between the reviewers and the PI
- Provide a means for the applicants to submit information that should have been in the application originally

- Provide a forum for debating priority score ratings in the absence of evidence of flawed reviews
- Reverse funding decisions

The new process consists of two potentially sequential phases.

Communication

In the first phase, the communications (rebuttals) are handled by program and review staff. Usually applicant investigators, who have concerns, will feel strongly about them and submit a letter of rebuttal. The letter should be addressed to the institute program administrator, if known. If not, it can be sent to the SRA.

The items in contention should be stated clearly and the rebuttal documented. Avoid being overly argumentative and engaging in personal attacks. It is important to remember that the actual and official applicant is your organization. In effect, when you communicate with NIH regarding your proposal, you are speaking on behalf of your organization.

The NIH component that is responsible for the application at the time the communication is received is also responsible for examining the concerns and responding to them. Thus, DRG is responsible for all issues relating to acceptance and assignment and the pending review by a DRG study section. After the initial review has been completed, the assigned funding institute is responsible. However, there will be considerable discussion and consultation between program and review staffs.

If it is determined that the assignment is correct, no change will be made. If no flaws in the review were identified, the recommendation to the PI will be to revise the proposal and resubmit.

If a serious flaw is found, the SRA, after consultation with the program administrator and with the approval of the review section chief, most likely will administratively defer the application. It will be brought back for rereview either by the same study section or by another appropriate review group. If the program and review staff persons cannot agree on a course of action, the rebuttal may be presented to the advisory council. In some institutes, all rebuttals in which the staff and the PI disagree are taken to the council. The council may recommend a project site visit, a rereview of the application, or concurrence with the study section action. If an applicant is dissatisfied with the decision on a rebuttal letter, a second, more formal avenue of appeal is available.

Appeals

The investigator may submit a formal appeal, which must be endorsed by the applicant institution. (The signature of the appropriate institutional official is required.) Some institutions may be reluctant to enter into this time-consuming process and obtaining an endorsement may not always be accomplished easily. However, if there is a strong case and the PI perseveres, the endorsed appeal, once submitted, becomes the responsibility of the NIH Appeals Officer, located in the Office of the Deputy Director for Extramural Research (DDER), NIH. At this point, any further consideration of the application will normally be interrupted until the issue is resolved. Also, if the proposal is revised and resubmitted while the appeal is pending, the original application will be inactivated and the appeal process ended.

The NIH Appeals Officer will notify the appropriate ICD, which will gather information to evaluate the appeal with the help of program and review staff. Usually, a committee of experts will be convened to review the documentation. These materials and the committee's recommendation are jointly examined by the DDER and the relevant ICD director(s), who will render a judgment and determine the proper course of action for the NIH. The options for resolution are the same as for resolving concerns expressed in a communication, i.e., no intervention, administrative deferral for rereview, or special council consideration. The decision is final and binding. An appeal does not guarantee the right to a reassignment, rereview, or special consideration of an application. In no case will the immediate outcome of an appeal be to fund. For further information, contact:

NIH Appeals Officer
Building 31, Room 5B31
National Institutes of Health
Bethesda, MD 20892
(301) 496–5358

13

Areas of Special Interest

Shared responsibility between members of the biomedical research community and NIH staff is an important aspect of the extramural programs and the peer review system. One aspect of this is service by members of the research community on advisory councils and review panels. In addition, many of these individuals are PIs themselves. They and their institutions as applicants share important roles in assuring the responsible and ethical conduct of research and the training for this, the proper care of human subjects and experimental animals in research protocols, the equitable involvement of minorities and women as subjects in clinical research, and the protection of research personnel and the environment.

HUMAN SUBJECTS

The official regulations of the DHHS on the protection of human subjects are spelled out in the *Code of Federal Regulations 45 CFR 46* (Department of Health and Human Services, 1983). However, the relevant rules and regulations are included in the instructions for all application forms. It is important to remember that it is possible for an application to be recommended for no further consideration if unethical practices, which carry risk of harm, are judged to be involved or be deferred if incomplete information is provided. Because of the length of time involved in the process, PIs should complete their applications in sufficient time for the appropriate institutional committees, which only meet periodically, to approve protocols involving human subjects.

Public Health Service policy requires that an Institutional Review Board (IRB) have at least five members with varied professional or vocational backgrounds (racial and cultural), experience, and expertise. The board should be sensitive to such issues as community attitudes and promoting respect for its own advice and counsel in safeguarding the rights and welfare of human subjects.

The membership should include individuals having the professional competence to review specific research activities. If an IRB regularly reviews research that involves vulnerable subjects such as children, prisoners, pregnant women, or handicapped or mentally disabled persons, its membership should include individuals knowledgeable about and experienced in working with these subjects. It may not consist entirely of men, entirely of women, or entirely of members of one profession. It is to include at least one nonscientific member and one member not affiliated with the institution and not part of the immediate family of one who is affiliated with the institution. Conflict of interest rules apply, and individuals with special expertise may be invited to assist in the review of complex issues on an ad hoc basis.

The IRB, in its review, can approve, require modifications to, or disapprove research activities involving human subjects. Experiments with human subjects must be designed to consider ethical and safety issues as well as to uncover new scientific knowledge. Thus, to approve the human subjects protocols, the IRB must be assured that risks to subjects are minimized and that the risks are reasonable in relation to the anticipated benefits and the importance of the knowledge to be gained. Further, the board will want to know that the selection of subjects is equitable, that informed consent will be sought and appropriately documented, and that there will be adequate monitoring of data collected to assure the safety of subjects. Additional assurances sought are that the privacy of patients will be protected and that safeguards will be in place to prevent coercion of, or undue influence on, subjects such as those with severe physical or mental illness or persons who are economically or educationally disadvantaged. For more information, contact:

> **Office for Protection from Research Risks**
> **Building 31, Room 5B59**
> **NIH**
> **Bethesda, MD 20892**
> **(301) 496–7005**

There are at least four places in the PHS 398 where the PI must pay attention if human subjects are involved in the proposal

Face Page

Item 4 must be completed if activities involving human subjects are planned at any time, whether or not exempt from the regulations. If exemptions apply, insert the exemption number(s) in the space provided. The activities that are exempt are listed in the General Information section of the instructions to the PHS 398 and include such things as educational tests (cognitive, diagnostic, aptitude, achievement), observations, and clinical materials where individuals cannot be identified. If the planned research protocols are not exempt, the assurance identification number must be inserted in 4b (if the applicant institution has a Multiple Project Assurance of Compliance on file with the Office for Protection from Research Risks [OPRR] of NIH).

The date of the IRB approval in item 4a must not be more than one year prior to the receipt date for which the application is being submitted. If approval has not been obtained, mark "pending" in that space and submit the follow-up certification of IRB approval within sixty days after the receipt date. It is the responsibility of the PI to get the certification to the SRA of the assigned review group in time. There may be no reminder to do so. If there is no assurance filed, insert "none" in 4b. The signed application signifies that there will be compliance and that this will be established within thirty days after the request from OPRR.

Budget

If there will be patient care costs related to the research, the clinical facilities to be used must be named and the basis for the costs provided unless there has been a DHHS-negotiated patient care rate agreement with the facility. Physician fees should be listed under Consultant Costs. Clinical costs for consortium or contractual organizations should be inserted under that category on the budget page. Travel, lodging, and subsistence costs for patients should be listed under Other Expenses.

Resources and Environment

The capacities and capabilities of the clinical facilities to be used should be indicated. Indicate the proximity to the main research facility as well as the frequency of availability to the investigative team.

Text

Here the PI has the opportunity and responsibility to describe the clinical protocols in detail. After the Section 4 on "Research Design and Methods", section 5, "Human Subjects," must address six points, the details of which are provided in the PHS 398 instructions and in Chapter 5, "Application Preparation."

Women and Minorities as Subjects

NIH policy states that research involving human subjects should be of benefit to all persons at risk of the disease or the condition regardless of gender or race. However, various task forces organized to study women's and minorities' health issues have noted gaps in the knowledge about these populations. They have been underrepresented in research studies, and there are clear scientific and public health reasons for specifically including them in study populations. Thus, applications involving human subjects must give appropriate attention to the inclusion of women and minorities in study populations. Principal investigators must supply clear and compelling reasons for not doing so unless it can be shown that including them would be impossible or inappropriate with respect to the purpose of the research or the health of the subjects. Also, if in the only study population available there is a disproportionate representation of one gender or minority group, the reasons for excluding one group or another must be well explained and justified.

If the application does not contain the necessary information, the assigned SRA will request written clarification. Failure of the PI to respond to this request will result in deferral or return of the application. In the case of responses to RFAs with single receipt dates, if PIs fail to comply with the review staff's requests for the information, the application will be returned without review. Underrepresented U.S. racial/ethnic minority populations include American Indians, Alaskan natives, Asian/Pacific Islanders, blacks, and Hispanics.

In all applications, the PI must describe the anticipated gender and racial/ethnic makeup of the study population. This information should be included in the Research Plan (items 1–4) of the application and summarized under Human Subjects (item 5). A study design should be employed with gender representation appropriate to the known incidence or prevalence of the condition being studied. Whenever there are scientific reasons to anticipate differences between men and women with regard to the hypothesis being studied, the PI should include an evaluation of gender and minority group differences in the proposed study.

Applicants should be aware that review panels, in evaluating applications, will be instructed to determine:

If sufficient attention has been paid to the inclusion of minorities, if there is an adequate number of women in the study design, and whether these considerations affect the ability to answer the scientific questions posed. A weakness or deficiency here could affect the outcome of the review negatively.

The compelling nature of the justification given by the PI for including only one minority group, only male subjects, or a study population with numbers of women not reflecting the gender prevalence of the condition under study. Funding will not be provided without such justification.

It is possible that the ethnic makeup or gender composition of the subjects involved will not be described because the PI did not perceive the need to include either in the study population. However, if the reviewers determine that the study has the potential to answer relevant scientific questions and translate the findings to all persons at risk, this will be documented by the SRA in the summary statement. No funding will be given until the applicant provides sufficient information on the study population to assure compliance with the policy. Thus, it pays to plan ahead to avoid delays in the processing of applications and the possible costly modification of research protocols. Publication of RFAs and PAs in the NIH Guide for Grants and Contracts will routinely include reminders of this issue.

Additionally, an Office of Research on Women's Health has been established at NIH to ensure the adequate representation of women in subject populations in research involving human subjects and to target research areas of particular concern to women. For more information, contact:

Office of Research on Women's Health
Building 1, Room 201
NIH
Bethesda, MD 20892
(301) 402–1770

VERTEBRATE ANIMALS

Policy (Office for Protection from Research Risks, 1986) requires that an Institutional Animal Care and Use Committee (IACUC) consist of no less than five members and include at least one doctor of veterinary medicine with training or experience in laboratory animal science and medicine, one practicing scientist experienced in research involving animals, one member from a nonscientific area, and one individual who is not affiliated with the institution and not a member of the immediate family of a person who is affiliated with the institution.

Among other things, it is the responsibility of an IACUC to review, at least once every six months, the institution's program for the humane care and use of animals and to inspect, at least once every six months, all of the institution's animal facilities. It must review and approve, require modifications in, or withhold approval of those components of USPHS-conducted or supported activities related to the care and use of animals. The IACUC also is authorized to suspend an activity involving animals, should a project be carried out contrary to the provisions of the Animal Welfare Act of 1966, as it is currently amended.

In reviewing the use of vertebrate animals in a research proposal, the IACUC must be assured that the procedures with animals will avoid or minimize discomfort, distress, and pain, that the procedures that may cause more than momentary or slight pain or distress will be performed with appropriate sedation, analgesia, or anesthesia, and that animals experiencing severe or chronic pain or distress that cannot be relieved will be painlessly sacrificed. The committee will want further assurances that the living conditions will be appropriate for the species of animal, that medical care will be available and provided for by a qualified veterinarian, that the personnel conducting the procedures will be appropriately trained and qualified, and that the methods of euthanasia used will be consistent with the recommendations of the American Veterinary Medical Association. For more information, contact:

Office for Protection from Research Risks
Building 31, Room 5B59
NIH
Bethesda, MD 20892
(301) 496–7005

Additionally, if vertebrate animals are to be used at any time in the research, NIH staff and the reviewers will evaluate the choice of species, the numbers to be employed, and whether the species are in short supply. They will review the costs, the care and maintenance of the animals, and the humane treatment to be used to reduce or minimize pain and suffering. As in the case of human subjects, there are a number of places in the PHS 398 where information on animals must be inserted.

Face Page

The proper information must be indicated in item 5. If the approval of the IACUC has not been obtained by submission time, "pending" should be inserted in 5a, and the signature of the institutional official on the bottom of the page assures that approval will be sought. Approval must be submitted within sixty days after the receipt date for which the application was submitted. The IACUC approval date must not be more than three years old.

Budget

In the Supplies category, indicate the number of animals to be used, their unit purchase cost, and unit care cost.

Resources and Environment

Animal facilities should be described, indicating their capacity, capabilities, proximity to the main research facility, and extent of availability to the proposed project.

Text

The protocols involving animals are detailed here. In addition, the five points required in section 6, Vertebrate Animals, must be completed. These are detailed in the PHS 398 instructions and in Chapter 5, "Application Preparation." Again, failure to include the necessary information will lead to a deferral of the review of the proposal.

BIOHAZARDS

Whether or not procedures, reagents, microorganisms, or other materials to be employed will be harmful to laboratory personnel or the environment is part of the review process. An application will not be recommended for further consideration or will be deferred if procedures or materials are judged to represent dangerous biohazards or if information provided is incomplete. For more information, contact:

Office for Protection from Research Risks
Building 31, Room 5B59
NIH
Bethesda, MD 20892
(301) 496–7005

MISCONDUCT IN SCIENCE

The DHHS has published regulations requiring the applicant institution to provide assurance that it has established policies and procedures for investigating and reporting instances of alleged or apparent scientific misconduct. Form PHS 6315, Initial Assurance Form, must be submitted to assure compliance.

If there are allegations of misconduct or fraud involving the PI of an application pending review, the study section will not be informed by staff and will carry out the review in the usual manner. However, it is possible that an application will be deferred if major allegations and questions regarding the PI or the institution become known. For more information, contact:

Office of Research Integrity
Division of Research Integrity Assurance
OASH, DHHS
Building 31, Room B1C39
NIH
Bethesda, MD 20892
(301) 496–2624

DRUG-FREE WORKPLACE

Before an award can be made, the applicant organization must certify that it will provide a drug-free workplace. The organization must:

- Publish a statement notifying employees that it is unlawful to manufacture controlled substances in the workplace and that the distribution, possession, or use of these substances is prohibited in the workplace. The action to be taken, if the prohibition is violated, must be specified.
- Establish a drug-awareness program
- Provide a copy of the statement to each employee participating in the grant
- Notify the employee that the condition of employment requires abiding by the terms of the statement
- Notify the USPHS-awarding unit of any employee convicted of a drug violation occurring in the workplace
- Require any employee so convicted to participate in a rehabilitation program

This information is located on the second page of the Checklist.

CONFLICT OF INTEREST

There is much concern over the appearance of a conflict of interest when drug development and testing studies are carried out. Principal investigators should be sensitive to their relationships with the government and the use of public funds for the research, to their institutions which receive the money, and to the more circumscribed interests of commercial organizations for which they may be consultants. Further, PIs are encouraged not to ask colleagues who are consultants to commercial organizations that could gain advantages from their research to participate in their proposed projects. Regulations currently are being formulated by DHHS to guide investigators in avoiding conflict of interest situations in this area.

RESPONSIBLE CONDUCT OF RESEARCH

Congress is concerned over allegations and reports of improper activities in research, especially that funded by the federal government. This has led to the revision of the guidelines for the submission of all competing Institutional Training Grant (T32) applications. It is required that some type of program on the principles of scientific integrity be an integral part of the proposed training effort. The grant application must include a description of the formal or informal activities the applicant organization will conduct to teach trainees ethical and scientifically responsible conduct in research. No award will be made until such a description is furnished.

14

Valuable Sources of Information

There is an abundance of information about the NIH extramural programs. This chapter makes reference to some but not all available materials. More information can be obtained by contacting an Office of Sponsored Research at your institution, the ICD information offices listed at the end of the chapter, or from the NIH staff.

Offices of Sponsored Research, or their equivalent, in applicant institutions can offer a variety of often overlooked services to assist in application submissions and in acquiring helpful information about NIH programs and those of other agencies. Also, the administrators of these offices are usually in a position to refer those seeking support to senior, knowledgeable investigators within the institution who have had experience with the NIH review and award process. These offices usually have application kits, brochures, and other references to federally sponsored programs.

The NIH offers a large number of informative publications describing various facets of the extramural programs. The most useful are highlighted below, together with the name of the office to contact to obtain copies. These publications and other sources of information are valuable to either investigators or administrators at institutions competing for grant and contract support.

NIH GUIDE FOR GRANTS AND CONTRACTS

This weekly publication is the best source of information about new PAs, RFAs, RFPs, and new or modified NIH extramural policy and administrative matters. It includes information about the programs of other Public Health Service agencies as well, such as the Food and Drug Administration. The material in each issue is usually arranged into several categories.

Notices

This section contains announcements of new or changes in extramural policies and procedures, conferences, workshops, and so forth.

Notices of Availability (RFPs and RFAs)

This section briefly states the objectives of RFAs for grants and cooperative agreements and RFPs, together with the name, address, and phone number of the staff member to contact for copies of the announcement or more information. In the case of some RFAs, the full announcement is provided.

Ongoing Program Announcements

This section identifies areas of special program interest for which grant applications are encouraged.

To get on the *Guide* mailing list, request a form from:

> **Printing and Reproduction Branch**
> **Building 31, Room B4BN08**
> **NIH**
> **Bethesda, MD 20892**
> **(301) 496–1787**

To receive a copy electronically, contact:

> **E-Guide**
> **Institutional Liaison Office**
> **Building 31, Room 5B31**
> **NIH**
> **Bethesda, MD 20892**
> **(301) 496–5366**

OFFICE OF GRANT INQUIRIES, DRG

This office is a very responsive, excellent information resource. It prepares and distributes numerous documents describing the extramural programs and has videocassettes available for loan. Also, it will supply single copies of application kits. The titles of the office's program guidelines, publications, and videocassettes are listed below.

Program Guidelines

Detailed information about the following grant programs is available:

NIH National Research Service Award—Institutional Grants (T32) Guidelines
NIH National Research Service Award—Senior Fellows (F33) Guidelines

NIH National Research Service Award—Individual Postdoctoral Fellows (F32) Guidelines

NIH National Research Service Award—Short-Term Training for Students in Health Professional Schools (T35) Guidelines

First Independent Research Support and Transition (FIRST) Award (R29) Guidelines

Guidelines for Establishing and Operating Consortium Grants

Support of Scientific Meetings (R13)

Small Grants Program (R03)

NIH Research Grants to Foreign Institutions and International Organizations

The K Awards—Research Career Program Awards

Academic Research Enhancement Award (AREA) (R15)

Publications

Information from the NIH on Grants and Contracts

This brochure lists available program guidelines and publications, most of which are noted in this chapter.

NIH Peer Review of Research Grant Applications

This is a booklet containing information on the peer review process, including tables and charts.

Helpful Hints on Preparing a Research Grant Application to the National Institutes of Health

Helpful Hints on Preparing a Fellowship Application to the National Institutes of Health

Peer Review Notes

This newsletter is published three times a year prior to review committee meetings. The purpose is to inform NIH consultants and staff about issues related to review policies and procedures.

NIH Extramural Programs—Funding for Research and Research Training

This booklet provides a brief description of the program interests and mechanisms of support offered by each awarding unit.

NIH Grants and Awards

This is a summary of the support mechanisms used by each of the awarding units.

Preparing a Research Grant Application to the National Institute of Health: Selected Articles

This is a bound collection of reprints with topics related to the peer review system and application preparation.

NIH Programs of Special Interest to Minorities

DRG Organization and Function

This brochure outlines the organization, functions, and staff, including names, addresses, and phone numbers of supervisors, referral officers, SRAs, and study sections.

Grants Administration Information Sources

This booklet lists NIH program and grant administrators, along with phone numbers.

Public Health Service Grants Policy Statement

This booklet states policies and issues relating to the administration of PHS grant awards. Single copies are available.

Videocassettes

The Peer Review System

How to Apply for an NIH Research Grant

How to Review a Research Grant

DRG Organization and Function

To obtain copies of the above documents, more information about the extramural programs, or to arrange for the loan of a videocassette, write or call:

> **Office of Grants Inquiries, DRG**
> **Room 449, Westwood Building**
> **NIH**
> **Bethesda, MD 20892**
> **(301) 496–7441**
> **(301) 496–9975 (FAX)**

OFFICE FOR PROTECTION FROM RESEARCH RISKS

Protection of Human Subjects

Federal regulations governing the protection of human subjects involved in research are described.

Also available are policy statements and regulations governing the protection of animals.

Office for Protection from Research Risks
Building 31, Room B59
NIH
Bethesda, MD 20892
(301) 496–8101 (Human Subjects)
(301) 496–7163 (Animal Welfare)

SMALL BUSINESS INNOVATION RESEARCH SOLICITATION OFFICE

Omnibus Solicitation of the Public Health Service for Small Business Innovation Research (SBIR)

Describes the program and includes SBIR grant application and guidelines.

Omnibus Solicitation of the Public Health Service for Small Business Innovation Research (SBIR)

This booklet describes guidelines for contract proposals.

For copies of these publications, write to:

SBIR Solicitation Office
13687 Baltimore Ave.
Laurel, MD 20707-5083
(301) 206–9385

For information about the SBIR program, write to:

Special Programs Officer
Building 31, Room 5B44
Bethesda, MD 20892
(301) 496–1968

ICD PUBLIC INQUIRIES OFFICES

Selected publications of interest prepared by the ICDs are noted below. In addition, these offices have available a large number of disease-oriented pamphlets and brochures, e.g., *Diabetes* (NIDDK), *Hypertension* (NHLBI), etc. If an address does not appear next to the publication, refer to the list of ICD Public Inquiries Offices in this chapter.

NATIONAL INSTITUTES OF HEALTH

NIH Data Book

This booklet contains interesting data on NIH extramural programs and other aspects of the NIH programs and staff.

> **Economics and Resources Studies Branch**
> **Division of Planning and Evaluation**
> **Office of Science Policy and Legislation**
> **Building 31, Room 4B35**
> **NIH**
> **Bethesda, MD 20892**
> **(301) 496–9285**

Research and Research Related Manpower Development Programs Supported by the National Institutes of Health

This is a summary of the research and training opportunities both extramurally and intramurally spanning all levels from high school to postdoctoral training.

> **Research Training and Special Programs Officer**
> **Office of Extramural Research**
> **Building 31, Room 5B44**
> **NIH**
> **Bethesda, MD 20892**
> **(301) 496–9743**

A Guide to the NIH Research Contracting Process

> **Division of Contracts and Grants**
> **Office of the Director**
> **Building 31, Room 1B03**
> **NIH**
> **Bethesda, MD 20892**
> **(301) 496–4422**

DIVISION OF RESEARCH GRANTS

The following booklets can be obtained by calling or writing to:

> **Information Systems Branch**
> **Westwood Building, Room 109**
> **NIH**
> **Bethesda, MD 20892**
> **(301) 496–7400**

Activity Codes, Organizational Codes, and Definitions Used in Extramural Programs

DRG Peer Review Trends

This is a two-volume set, one of which provides workload and review data of DRG study sections and ICD review committees. The other highlights characteristics of advisory committee members such as educational background, age, rank, women, and minorities.

NIH Extramural Trends

This booklet presents data on extramural awards.

IMPAC: A Computer Based Information System for the Extramural Programs of NIH/PHS

This booklet describes the data system used for the extramural programs.

CRISP: What Is the CRISP System?

CRISP is the acronym for Computer Retrieval of Information on Scientific Projects, which supplies research data on funded extramural awards organized according to scientific areas.

NIH Research Grants (Vol. 1); R & D Contracts, Grants for Training, Construction, and Medical Libraries (Vol. 2)

These booklets list grants and awards funded during FY 1989 by geographic area, organization, and principal investigator.

NATIONAL INSTITUTE ON AGING

Funding Facts: Grants and Contracts

This describes the institute's programs and awards.

National Institute on Aging Research Training and Career Opportunities

Describes the institute's extramural and intramural award opportunities.

NATIONAL INSTITUTE OF GENERAL MEDICAL SCIENCES

The following provide excellent data and descriptions of the institute's programs.

Biophysics and Physiological Sciences Program

Cellular and Molecular Basis of Disease Program

Genetics Program

Pharmacological Sciences Program

Grant Award Mechanisms

Minority Biomedical Research Support Program

Minority Access to Research Careers (MARC) Program

Medical Scientist Training Program

NATIONAL HEART, LUNG, AND BLOOD INSTITUTE

National Heart, Lung, and Blood Institute Program Project Grant, Preparation of an Application

Describes the concept, characteristics, and instructions for preparation of applications.

National Heart, Lung, and Blood Institute Guidelines for Demonstration and Education Research Grants

Provides information for investigators interested in applying for demonstration and education grants.

NATIONAL INSTITUTE OF ENVIRONMENTAL HEALTH SCIENCES

National Institute of Environmental Health Sciences Research Programs

NATIONAL INSTITUTE OF NEUROLOGICAL DISORDERS AND STROKE

NINDS Extramural Research and Training Awards

JOHN E. FOGARTY INTERNATIONAL CENTER

John E. Fogarty International Center—Opportunities in Biomedical Research

NATIONAL CENTER FOR NURSING RESEARCH

National Center for Nursing Research: Facts About Funding

NATIONAL CENTER FOR RESEARCH RESOURCES

Biomedical Research Support Shared Instrumentation Grant Program Folder

ICD Public Inquiries Offices

Office	Address	Telephone
OD/NIH	Building 31, Room 2B03	(301) 496–4143
DRG	Westwood Bldg., Room 449	(301) 496–7441
NCRR	Building 12A, Room 4007	(301) 496–5795
FIC	Building 31, Room B2C29	(301) 496–2075
NCI	Building 31, Room 10A29	(301) 496–6631
NCNR	Building 31, Room 5B25	(301) 496–0207
NEI	Building 31, Room 6A32	(301) 496–5248
NHLBI	Building 31, Room 4A21	(301) 496–4236
NIAID	Building 31, Room 7A32	(301) 496–5717
NIAMS	Building 31, Room 4C05	(301) 496–8188
NICHD	Building 31, Room 2A34	(301) 496–5133
NIDCD	Building 31, Room 3C35	(301) 496–7243
NIDR	Building 31, Room 2C33	(301) 496–4261
NIDDK	Building 31, Room 9A04	(301) 496–3583
NIEHS	P.O. Box 12233 Research Triangle Park, NC 27709	(919) 629–3345
NIGMS	Building 31, Room 4A52	(301) 496–7301
NINDS	Building 31, Room 8A16	(301) 496–5751
NIA	Building 31, Room 5C27	(301) 496–1752
NLM	Building 38, Room 2S10	(301) 496–6308
NCHGR	Building 38A, Room 615	(301) 402–0911

Biomedical Research Technology Program—Guidelines, Application, and Instructions

Guide for the Care and Use of Laboratory Animals

ICD PUBLIC INQUIRIES OFFICE

Correspondence should be directed to the "Public Inquiries Office" at each institute in the accompanying chart. All addresses should conclude with Bethesda, MD 20892, except as noted.

Appendix 1

Instructions for PHS 398
Rev. 9/91

Form Approved Through 6/30/94
OMB No. 0925-0001

U.S. DEPARTMENT OF HEALTH
AND HUMAN SERVICES
Public Health Service

GRANT APPLICATION FORM PHS 398

I. THE PHS PEER REVIEW PROCESS

The application that you submit to the Public Health Service (PHS) will be reviewed through a dual system, in which the first level of review will be performed by an Initial Review Group (IRG), often called a Study Section, and the second level of review will usually be performed by the Advisory Council or Board of the potential awarding component (Institute, Center, or other unit, hereafter referred to as Institute). There are some programs where the second review is other than by Council or Board, and this process is described in applicable program announcements.

Most grant applications submitted to the various agencies of the PHS must be submitted through the Referral Section, Division of Research Grants (DRG), National Institutes of Health (NIH). This includes applications intended not only for the NIH, but also for the Alcohol, Drug Abuse, and Mental Health Administration (ADAMHA), Food and Drug Administration (FDA), Agency for Health Care Policy and Research (AHCPR), Health Resources and Services Administration (HRSA), and Centers for Disease Control (CDC).

Within the DRG Referral Section, administrative information about the application is entered into the computer system. The application is then assigned to the most appropriate IRG or Study Section for a scientific merit review. Assignments are based on the scientific content of the entire application, including the specific aims, methodology, and overall focus. The assignment criteria are specified in DRG and IRG Institute referral guidelines. Applications are also assigned to the appropriate PHS agency, where most will receive a second level, programmatic review by the Advisory Council or Board of an Institute. Assignments are made by Referral Officers. These individuals are professional scientists, most of whom also serve as Scientific Review Administrators of DRG Study Sections.

For most applications, the minimum time from receipt to award is approximately 10 months. The initial scientific merit review generally takes place within 4 months of receipt, after which the results for most applications recommended for further consideration are conveyed to Institute Advisory Councils in a summary statement. A copy of this summary statement is usually sent by the Institute to the investigator about 1 month before the Council meets. Councils generally meet 3 or 4 months after the initial review, and awards are made after the Council has met.

More information about the PHS peer review system and specific grant programs can be obtained from the DRG Office of Grants Inquiries at (301)496-7441. Information about charters and membership of Public Advisory Groups (IRGs, Study Sections, and Institute Councils) can be obtained from the appropriate agencies.

Applicants should be aware of the availability of presubmission advice from staff of the Institute to which an application may be assigned. Because Institute staff can provide helpful comments and advice regarding the general approach taken in preparing an application, applicants are **encouraged** to contact staff of the relevant Institute. Initial contact points for staff of the various agencies or Institutes within the PHS are listed below:

3

AWARDING COMPONENTS OF THE
PUBLIC HEALTH SERVICE

AGENCY	INSTITUTE	CONTACT/PHONE
Agency for Health Care Policy and Research (AHCPR)		(301)443-5650
Alcohol, Drug Abuse, and Mental Health Administration (ADAMHA)	Office of the Administrator	(301)443-4266
ADAMHA	National Institute on Alcohol Abuse and Alcoholism	(301)443-4375
ADAMHA	National Institute on Drug Abuse	(301)443-2755
ADAMHA	National Institute of Mental Health	(301)443-3367
ADAMHA	Office for Substance Abuse Prevention	(301)443-0365
ADAMHA	Office of Treatment Improvement	(301)443-9923
Food and Drug Administration (FDA)		(301)443-6170
Centers for Disease Control (CDC)	National Institute for Occupational Safety and Health	(404)639-3343
National Institutes of Health (NIH)	National Institute on Aging	(301)496-9322
NIH	National Institute of Allergy and Infectious Diseases	(301)496-7291
NIH	National Institute of Arthritis and Musculoskeletal and Skin Diseases	(301)496-0802
NIH	National Cancer Institute	(301)496-7173
NIH	National Institute of Child Health and Human Development	(301)496-1485
NIH	National Institute on Deafness and Other Communication Disorders	(301)496-1804
NIH	National Institute of Dental Research	(301)496-6324
NIH	National Institute of Diabetes and Digestive and Kidney Diseases	(301)496-7277
NIH	National Institute of Environmental Health Sciences	(919)541-7634
NIH	National Eye Institute	(301)496-5884
NIH	Fogarty International Center	(301)496-1653

4

NIH	National Institute of General Medical Sciences	(301)496-7061
NIH	National Heart, Lung, and Blood Institute	(301)496-7416
NIH	National Center for Human Genome Research	(301)496-7531
NIH	National Library of Medicine	(301)496-4621
NIH	National Institute of Neurological Disorders and Stroke	(301)496-9248
NIH	National Center for Nursing Research	(301)496-0523
NIH	National Center for Research Resources	(301)496-9971
Office of Population Affairs Office of the Assistant Secretary for Health (OASH)	Office of Family Planning	(202)245-0151
OASH	Office of Adolescent Pregnancy Programs	(202)245-7473

II. TYPES OF APPLICATIONS AND REQUIRED FORMS

Use Form PHS 398 to apply for all new, competing continuation, and supplemental research and research training grant and cooperative agreement support, except as shown in the table below:

Type of Application	Use Form Number
Small Business Innovation Research Program-Phase I	PHS 6246-1
Small Business Innovation Research Program-Phase II	PHS 6246-2
Individual National Research Service Award or Senior International Fellowship Award	PHS 416-1
International Research Fellowship Award	NIH 1541-1

In addition the following programs do not use the PHS 398:

Nonresearch Training Grant	PHS 6025
Health Services Project	PHS 5161-1

Most of the above application forms have corresponding forms to be used when applying for noncompeting continuation support during an approved project period. For Form PHS 398, the appropriate form for noncompeting continuation applications is Form PHS 2590.

The instructions provided in this kit pertain to applications for traditional, unsolicited, investigator-initiated, research project grants and cooperative agreements. Use the additional instructions and substitute pages included at the back of this kit when applying for a Research Career Development Award (K04) or an Institutional National Research Service Award. Request additional instructions from the PHS components indicated below when using Form PHS 398 to apply for other specialized grants. These include but are not limited to those listed below. *For these specialized grant applications, applicants are urged to consult with the appropriate PHS awarding component prior to submission.* Some of these grant applications use the regular receipt dates shown on page 8,

5

whereas others (indicated by an *) have special receipt dates as indicated. For further information, call the Office of Grants Inquiries, Division of Research Grants, NIH at (301)496-7441.

Academic Investigator Award (K07):
Appropriate component of the National Institutes of Health, Bethesda, MD 20892, or the Alcohol, Drug Abuse, and Mental Health Administration, Rockville, MD 20857.

*Academic Research Enhancement Award (AREA-R15):
Office of Grants Inquiries, Division of Research Grants, National Institutes of Health, Bethesda, MD 20892. One annual receipt date, usually June 22.

Animal Resources Grant (P40):
National Center for Research Resources, National Institutes of Health, Bethesda, MD 20892.

*Biomedical Research Support Grant (S07):
National Center for Research Resources, National Institutes of Health, Bethesda, MD 20892. One annual receipt date, usually late December.

Biomedical Research Technology Resource Grant (P41):
National Center for Research Resources, National Institutes of Health, Bethesda, MD 20892.

Clinical Investigator Award (K08):
Office of Grants Inquiries, Division of Research Grants, National Institutes of Health, Bethesda, MD 20892.

*Community Clinical Oncology Grant (U10):
National Cancer Institute, National Institutes of Health, Bethesda, MD 20892. One annual receipt date, August 24.

Conference Grant (R13):
Office of Grants Inquiries, Division of Research Grants, National Institutes of Health, Bethesda, MD 20892.

First Independent Research Support and Transition Award (FIRST-R29):
Office of Grants Inquiries, Division of Research Grants, National Institutes of Health, Bethesda, MD 20892, or the Alcohol, Drug Abuse, and Mental Health Administration, Rockville, MD 20857. **NOTE:** Three reference letters (in sealed envelopes) must be **attached** to the face page of the original application and submit-

ted with the application (new or revised). A letter or memorandum from a department head or dean should also be submitted with the application. In addition, list individuals submitting letters of reference. Provide the name, title, and institutional affiliation for each individual following Literature Cited in the Research Plan.

General Clinical Research Center Grant (M01):
National Center for Research Resources, National Institutes of Health, Bethesda, MD 20892.

Investigator-initiated Multicenter Clinical Trial Grant (U10):
Appropriate component of the National Institutes of Health, Bethesda, MD 20892.

Minority Access to Research Careers Training Grant (T34):
National Institute of General Medical Sciences, National Institutes of Health, Bethesda, MD 20892, or the Alcohol, Drug Abuse, and Mental Health Administration, Rockville, MD 20857.

Minority Biomedical Research Support Grant (S06):
National Institute of General Medical Sciences, National Institutes of Health, Bethesda, MD 20892.

*Minority School Faculty Development Award (K14):
National Heart, Lung, and Blood Institute, National Institutes of Health, Bethesda, MD 20892. One annual receipt date, April 1.

NLM Resource Improvement Grant (G07):
National Library of Medicine, National Institutes of Health, Bethesda, MD 20894.

*Outstanding Investigator Grant (R35):
National Cancer Institute, National Institutes of Health, Bethesda, MD 20892. One annual receipt date, varying from year to year.

Physician Scientist Award (K11):
Office of Grants Inquiries, Division of Research Grants, National Institutes of Health, Bethesda, MD 20892.

Program Project (P01) and Center Grants (P50):
Appropriate component of the National Institutes of Health, Bethesda, MD 20892, or the Alcohol, Drug Abuse, and Mental Health Administration, Rockville, MD 20857.

Publication Grant (R01):
National Library of Medicine, National Institutes of Health, Bethesda, MD 20894.

Research Scientist Development (K02) and Research Scientist Awards (K05):
Appropriate Institute of the Alcohol, Drug Abuse, and Mental Health Administration, Rockville, MD 20857.

Scientist Development Award for Clinicians (K20) and Scientist Development Award (K21):
Appropriate Institute of the Alcohol, Drug Abuse, and Mental Health Administration, Rockville, MD 20857.

*Shared Instrumentation Grant (S10):
National Center for Research Resources, National Institutes of Health, Bethesda, MD 20892. One annual receipt date, usually in March, can vary from year to year.

*Short-Term Training Grant for Students in Health Professional Schools (T35):
Office of Grants Inquiries, Division of Research Grants, National Institutes of Health, Bethesda, MD 20892. One annual receipt date, January 10.

*Small Research Grant (R03):
Office of Grants Inquiries, Division of Research Grants, National Institutes of Health, Bethesda, MD 20892, or the Alcohol, Drug Abuse, and Mental Health Administration, Rockville, MD 20857. Receipt dates vary depending on the funding component.

Special Emphasis Research Career Award (K01):
National Center for Research Resources, National Institutes of Health, Bethesda, MD 20892, or National Institute on Aging, Bethesda, MD 20892.

*PROGRAM ANNOUNCEMENTS/REQUESTS FOR APPLICATIONS
When responding to a specific program announcement (PA) or request for applications (RFA) published in the *NIH Guide for Grants and Contracts*, the *Federal Register*, or other public media, contact the issuing PHS component for additional instructions.

III. SUBMISSION AND ASSIGNMENT

Mail or deliver the complete and signed, typewritten original of the application and five signed,

exact, clear, single-sided photocopies, in one package with the appendices, to the Division of Research Grants, National Institutes of Health, Room 240, Westwood Building, 5333 Westbard Avenue, Bethesda, MD 20892. This zip code is for central receipt of NIH mail. Applicants who wish to use express mail or a courier service should change the zip code to 20816.

Secure the application and its copies with rubber bands or paper clips **only**. Submit the Personal Data form with the original application, not with the copies. The application package must contain the original and copies of only one application. Do not submit different grant applications in the same package.

Simultaneous submissions of identical applications to different agencies within the PHS, or to different Institutes within an agency will not be allowed, nor will essentially identical applications be reviewed by the same or different review committees. Exceptions to this are: 1) individuals submitting an application for a Research Career Development Award who may propose essentially identical research in an application for an individual research project, and 2) individuals who may submit an individual research project essentially identical to a subproject that is part of a Program Project or Center grant application.

Submit a complete application. **An application will be considered incomplete and returned if it is illegible, if it fails to follow the instructions, or if the material presented is insufficient to permit an adequate review.** Unless specifically required by these instructions (e.g., human subjects certification, vertebrate animals verification, changes in other support), do **not** send supplementary or corrective material pertinent to an application after the receipt date without its being specifically solicited or agreed to by prior discussion with the Scientific Review Administrator of the IRG. Because there is no guarantee that the reviewers will consider late material, it is **essential** that the application be complete and accurate at the time of submission.

The PHS uses the following receipt, review, and award schedule:

7

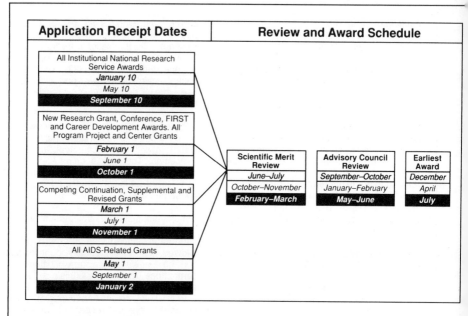

Application Receipt Dates	Review and Award Schedule

All Institutional National Research Service Awards
- January 10
- May 10
- September 10

New Research Grant, Conference, FIRST and Career Development Awards. All Program Project and Center Grants
- February 1
- June 1
- October 1

Competing Continuation, Supplemental and Revised Grants
- March 1
- July 1
- November 1

All AIDS-Related Grants
- May 1
- September 1
- January 2

Scientific Merit Review	Advisory Council Review	Earliest Award
June–July	September–October	December
October–November	January–February	April
February–March	May–June	July

January 2, May 1, and September 1, have been established as receipt dates for all investigator-initiated Acquired Immune Deficiency Syndrome (AIDS) research grant applications. These receipt dates have been established in order to accomplish the receipt-to-award process in an accelerated fashion, as mandated by law. These receipt dates are for *all* new, revised, competing continuation, and supplemental AIDS applications.

Applications will be considered to be "on time" if they are either (1) received on or before the established deadline date or (2) sent on or before the established deadline date and received in time for orderly processing. (Applicants should request a legibly dated U.S. Postal Service postmark or obtain a legibly dated receipt from a commercial carrier or the U.S. Postal Service. Private metered postmarks shall not be acceptable as proof of timely mailing.) If the receipt date falls on a weekend, it will be extended to the following Monday; if the date falls on a holiday, it will be extended to the following work day. The receipt date will be waived only in extenuating circumstances. To request such a waiver, include an explanatory letter with the signed, completed application. **No request for a waiver will be considered prior to receipt of the application, and there is no guarantee that the waiver will be granted.**

When submitting an application, the principal investigator/program director may suggest up to three IRGs and/or a PHS component to which it could be appropriately assigned. These suggestions will be taken into consideration at the time of assignment, although the final determination will be made by the PHS. However, do not send such correspondence under separate cover; attach it to the application at the time of submission.

As soon as possible after the receipt date, usually within 6 weeks, the PHS will send the principal investigator/program director and the applicant organization the application's assigned number and the name, address, and telephone number of the Scientific Review Administrator of the IRG to which it has been assigned, as well as the assigned Institute contact and phone number. If this information is **not** received within that time, contact the Referral Office, Division of Research Grants, National Institutes of Health, Bethesda,

8

MD 20892, Telephone: (301)496-7447. If there is a change in assignment, another notification is sent to the principal investigator/program director.

Once the assignment has been made, the principal investigator/program director may request reassignment if the initial assignment seems inappropriate. Such requests should be made in writing to the Referral Office, Division of Research Grants, National Institutes of Health, Westwood Building, Rm. 248, Bethesda, MD 20892. Although these requests will be carefully considered, again, the final determination will be made by the PHS.

IV. PREPARATION OF THE APPLICATION

A. GENERAL INSTRUCTIONS

Read and follow the instructions carefully to avoid delays and misunderstandings. Before preparing an application, review the Public Health Service Grants Policy Statement generally available in your institutional research grant administrative office. Specific program announcements (PAs) and requests for applications (RFAs) are published in the *Federal Register* and in the *NIH Guide for Grants and Contracts*. The *Guide* also contains vital information about policies and procedures and is being transmitted electronically to a number of institutions. To obtain the *Guide* on a regular basis, have your name included on the mailing list by contacting the Office of Grants Inquiries, Division of Research Grants, National Institutes of Health, Bethesda, MD 20892.

In preparing the application, use English only and avoid jargon. For terms not universally known, spell out the term the first time it is used with the appropriate abbreviation in parentheses; the abbreviation may be used thereafter. Type the application, single spaced, and stay within the margin limitations indicated on the form and continuation pages. Do not type in the shaded spaces; the type must be clear and legible. Use standard size black type (see page 10) that can be copied; do **not** use photoreduction. Draw all graphs, diagrams, tables, and charts in black ink. Do **not** include glossy photographs or other materials that cannot be copied in the body of the

application; submit them in five collated sets in the appendix. See further instructions on page 24 and in the appendix.

Computer-generated facsimiles may be substituted for any of the forms provided in this packet. Such substitute forms should be printed in black ink, but they must maintain the exact wording and format of the government-printed forms, including all captions and spacing. Any deviation may be grounds for the PHS to reject the entire application. Two copies of each form page are provided in this application. Form pages have also been printed individually, and copies are available from the applicant's office of sponsored research or from the Division of Research Grants, NIH.

Page limitations must be observed for each section, or the application will be returned without review. A summary of the page and content limitations is given in the following chart:

Page Limitations and Content Requirements		
Section	Page Limit	Content
Introduction		
Revised applications	3	See instructions on page 19.
Supplemental applications	1	See instructions on page 19.
Research Plan Sections 1-4	25 (excluding publications listed in Progress Report)	Text plus all figures, charts, tables and diagrams
Biographical Sketches	2 each	One sketch of not more than two pages for **each** key person, collaborator and consultant
Literature Cited	6	Complete citations, including titles and **all** authors
Appendix	—	No more than 10 publications, including accepted or submitted manuscripts
		Photographs (include a copy in the Research Plan)
		Questionnaires
		Other materials which do not photocopy well

Only in cases involving interdependent multiple subprojects (e.g., Program Projects, Multi-Center Clinical Trials) will the PHS determine that applications exceeding the page limitations are acceptable. However, specific page limits may apply to each subproject. For information pertaining to page limits for such projects, contact the funding component to which the application may be assigned (see page 4). The page limitations may also be different for other specialized grant applications listed in the section entitled Types of Applications and Required Forms (page 5). For information regarding page limitations, request and follow the additional instructions for those applications. Any additional questions should be directed to the Referral Office, DRG at (301)496-7447.

Type size limitations must be observed throughout the application, or the application will be returned without review. For the face page, the type density must be 10 characters per inch (cpi). This limit is to assure that all data typed in this page can be captured for computer processing without truncation. For the rest of the application, the type must be **clear and readily legible**, standard size, which is 10 to 12 points (approximately 1/8 inch in height for capital letters). If constant spacing is used, there should be no more than 15 cpi, whereas proportional spacing should provide an *average* of no more than 15 cpi. Finally, there must be no more than six lines of text within a vertical inch. Figures, charts, tables, figure legends, and footnotes may be smaller in size but must be clear and readily legible. Applications not meeting these requirements will be returned without review, or may be subject to deferral.

B. SPECIFIC INSTRUCTIONS–Forms

(Form Page 1) Type in the **unshaded** areas only. Type density must be 10 cpi.

Item 1. Title of Project. Choose a title that is descriptive and specifically appropriate, rather than general. **Do not exceed 56 typewriter spaces, including the spaces between words and punctuation.** A **New** application must have a different title from any other PHS project with the same principal investigator/program director. A **Competing Continuation** or **Revised** application should ordinarily have the same title as the previous grant or application. If the specific aims of the project have changed significantly, choose a new title. A **Supplemental** application **must** have the same title as the currently funded grant.

Item 2a. Response to Specific Request for Applications (RFA) or Program Announcement (PA). If the application is submitted in response to a published specific RFA or PA, check the box marked "YES" and identify the number of the RFA or the number and title of the PA. The term "specific program announcement" also includes specialized grants, such as the First Independent Research Support and Transition Award, Research Career Development Award, Academic Research Enhancement Award, Institutional National Research Service Award, and those listed under "Types of Applications and Required Forms" beginning on page 5. Attach the RFA label, which is under the general mailing label, to the bottom of the face page of the original and place the original on top of the entire package.

Item 2b. Type of Grant Program. This list includes the more commonly sought types of grants. Enter the code that designates the grant program for which this application is being prepared. This may be obtained from the list below or may be indicated in a particular RFA or PA to which you are responding. If you are not certain which code matches the program you are interested in, select "Other Grant Program" (XXX).

Academic Investigator Award	K07
Academic Research Enhancement Award (AREA)	R15
Animal Resources Grant	P40
Biomedical Research Support Grant	S07
Biomedical Research Technology Resource Grant	P41
Center Core Grant	P30
Clinical Investigator Award	K08
Community Clinical Oncology Grant	U10
Comprehensive Center	P60
Conference Grant	R13
Dentist Scientist Award (Individual)	K15
First Independent Research Support and Transition Award (FIRST)	R29
General Clinical Research Center Grant	M01
Institutional National Research Service Award (Training Grant)	T32

Minority Access to Research Careers Training Grant	T34	Research Project (Cooperative Agreement)	U01
Minority Biomedical Research Support Grant	S06	Research Scientist Award	K05
Minority High School Student Research Apprentice Program	S03	Research Scientist Development Award	K02
		Resource-Related Project Grant	R24
NLM Resource Improvement Grant	G07	Scientist Development Award for Clinicians	K20
NLM Resource Project Grant	G08		
Outstanding Investigator Grant	R35	Scientist Development Award	K21
Physician Scientist Award (Individual)	K11	Shared Instrumentation Grant	S10
Physician Scientist Award (Institutional)	K12	Short-Term Training for Students in Health Professional Schools	T35
Program Project Grant	P01		
Regular (Individual Investigator) Research Grant	R01	Small Grant	R03
		Specialized Center Grant	P50
Research Career Development Award	K04	Other Grant Program (not identified above)	XXX
Research Demonstration and Dissemination Project	R18		

Item 3a. Name of Principal Investigator/Program Director. Name the *one* person responsible to the applicant organization for the scientific and technical direction of the project. The concept of co-principal investigator is not formally recognized and therefore, staff will conduct official business with the principal investigator or institutional official only. A supplemental application must have the same principal investigator/program director as the currently funded grant.

Item 3b. Degree(s). Indicate all academic and professional degrees, as well as other credentials, such as licenses (e.g., R.N.).

Item 3c. Social Security Number. The PHS requests the Social Security Number for the purpose of accurate identification, referral, and review of applications and for efficient management of PHS grant programs. Provision of the Social Security Number is voluntary. No individual will be denied any right, benefit, or privilege provided by law because of refusal to disclose his or her Social Security Number.

Item 3d. Position Title. If the principal investigator/program director has more than one title, indicate the one most relevant to the proposed project, such as Professor of Biochemistry, Chief of Surgical Service, or Group Leader.

Item 3e. Mailing Address. Use complete information necessary for postal delivery. All written communications with the principal investigator will use this address. If the principal investigator can receive electronic mail via BITNET or INTERNET, enter the appropriate electronic network address as the last line in this field.

Item 3f. Department, Service, Laboratory, or Equivalent. Indicate the organizational affiliation, such as Department of Medicine, Materials Research Laboratory, or Social Sciences Institute.

Item 3g. Major Subdivision. Indicate the school, college, or other major subdivision, such as medical, dental, engineering, graduate, nursing, or public health. If there is no such subdivision, enter "NONE."

Item 3h. Telephone and FAX Numbers. Use a daytime telephone where the principal investigator can be reached, and, if available, a FAX number.

Item 4. Human Subjects. The Federal regulations for the protection of human subjects define "human subject" as a "living individual about whom an investigator obtains (1) data through intervention or interaction with the individual, or (2) identifiable private information."

11

The regulations extend to the use of human organs, tissue and body fluids from individually identifiable human subjects as well as to graphic, written, or recorded information derived from individually identifiable human subjects. The use of autopsy materials is governed by applicable State and local law and is not directly regulated by the Federal human subject regulations.

If activities involving human subjects are not planned **at any time** during the proposed project period, check the box marked "NO" at Item 4a. The remaining parts of Item 4 are then not applicable.

If activities involving human subjects, whether or not exempt from Federal regulations for the protection of human subjects, are planned **at any time** during the proposed project period, either at the applicant organization or at any other performance site or collaborating institution, check the box marked "YES" at Item 4a. If the activities are designated to be exempt from the regulations, insert the exemption number(s) corresponding to one or more of the six exemption categories listed under Human Subjects in the Discussion of Assurance and Certification Requirements (Section E, page 25). The remaining parts of Item 4a are then not applicable. **Inappropriate designations of the non-involvement of human subjects or of exempt categories of research may result in delays in the review of an application. The PHS will make a final determination as to whether the proposed activities are covered by the regulations or are in an exempt category, based on the information provided in Section 5, page 22 of the Research Plan. In doubtful cases, prior consultation with the Office for Protection from Research Risks (OPRR), National Institutes of Health, Bethesda, MD 20892, Telephone: (301) 496-7041 is recommended.**

If the planned activities involving human subjects are not exempt, complete the remaining parts of Item 4a. If the applicant organization has an approved Multiple Project Assurance of Compliance on file with the OPRR that covers the specific activity, insert the Assurance identification number and the latest date of approval by the Institu-

tional Review Board (IRB) of the proposed activities. This date must be no earlier than one year before the receipt date for which the application is submitted. **This information in Items 4a and 4b and the signatures on the face page, as well as the assurance on the checklist, fulfill the requirement for certification of IRB approval.**

To ensure against delays in the review of the application, IRB review is best completed prior to submission of the application. However, if the IRB review is unavoidably delayed beyond the submission of the application, enter "pending" at Item 4a. A follow-up certification of IRB approval from an official signing for the applicant organization must then be sent to and received by the Scientific Review Administrator of the initial review group within 60 days after the receipt date for which the application is submitted. This follow-up certification format must include: application number, title of the application project, name of the principal investigator and institution, Multiple Project Assurance number, date of IRB approval, and appropriate signatures.

Any modifications in the Research Plan section of the application required by the IRB must be submitted with the follow-up certification. Occasionally PHS initial review may be scheduled to occur before the end of the 60-day grace period. In these special cases of accelerated review, the follow-up certification will be requested earlier. **Otherwise, it is the responsibility of the applicant organization to submit the follow-up certification. The PHS does not guarantee that it will remind the applicant organization or the principal investigator/program director to provide this missing information. If certification of IRB approval is not received when due, i.e., within 60 days after the official application receipt date, the application will be considered incomplete and deferred to the next review cycle.**

The name and address of the Scientific Review Administrator of the initial review group will be sent to the principal investigator/program director and applicant organization as soon as possible after the receipt date, usually within 6 weeks. To avoid delays in review, do not send the follow-up information to any other addresses. If the applicant organization does not have on file with OPRR an approved Assurance of Compliance, insert "NONE" in Item 4b. In this case, the applicant organization, by the signatures on the face page, is declaring that it will comply with 45 CFR 46 (the regulations for Protection of Human Subjects) by establishing an IRB and submitting an Assurance of Compliance and certification of IRB approval within 30 days of a specific request from OPRR.

An IRB of an institution with a Multiple Project Assurance of Compliance may review an application through an expedited review procedure provided it complies with the provisions of Section 46.110 of the human subject regulations 45 CFR 46. Check the type of review in the appropriate box on the checklist.

Item 5. Vertebrate Animals. If activities involving vertebrate animals are not planned **at any time** during the proposed project period, check the box marked "NO" at Item 5a. The remaining parts of Item 5 are then not applicable.

If activities involving vertebrate animals are planned **at any time** during the proposed project period, either at the applicant organization or at any other performance site or collaborating institution, check the box marked "YES" at Item 5a. If the applicant organization has an approved Animal Welfare Assurance on file with OPRR, insert at Item 5b the Assurance identification number and the date of approval by the Institutional Animal Care and Use Committee (IACUC) of those sections of the application related to the care and use of animals. **This information in Item 5a and 5b and the signatures on the face page fulfill the requirement for verification of IACUC approval.**

To ensure against delays in the review of the application, IACUC review is best completed prior to submission of the application. However, if the IACUC review is unavoidably delayed beyond the submission of the application, enter "pending" at Item 5b. A follow-up verification of IACUC approval from an official signing for the applicant organization must then be sent to and received by the Scientific Review Administrator of the initial review group within 60 days after the receipt date for which the application is submitted. This follow-up verification format must include: application number, title of application project, name of principal investigator and institution, Animal Welfare Assurance number, date of IACUC approval, and appropriate signatures.

Any modifications of the Research Plan section of the application required by the IACUC must be submitted with the follow-up verification. Occasionally PHS initial review may be scheduled to occur before the end of this 60-day grace period. In these special cases of accelerated review, the follow-up verification will be requested earlier. **Otherwise, it is the responsibility of the applicant organization to submit the follow-up verification. The PHS does not guarantee that it will remind the applicant organization or the principal investigator/program director to provide this missing information. If verification of IACUC approval is not received when due, i.e., within 60 days after the official application receipt date, the application will be considered incomplete and deferred to the next review cycle.**

The name and address of the Scientific Review Administrator of the initial review group will be sent to the principal investigator/program director and applicant organization as soon as possible after the receipt date, usually within 6 weeks. To avoid delays in review, do not send the follow-up information to any other addresses.

If the applicant organization does not have on file with OPRR an approved Animal Welfare Assurance, insert "NONE" in Item 5b. In this case, the applicant organization, by the signatures on the face page, is declaring that it will comply with PHS policy regarding the care and use of animals by establishing an IACUC and submitting an Animal Welfare Assurance and verification of IACUC approval when requested to do so by OPRR.

Item 6. Dates of Entire Proposed Project Period. Request no more than 5 years of support for the entire proposed project period; do not exceed 3 years for **Foreign** applicant organizations. To select an appropriate beginning date for a **New** or **Supplemental** application, consult the review and award schedule in these instructions on page 8. For a **Competing Continuation** application, choose a beginning date immediately

13

following the termination date of the current project period. Submit a **Supplemental** application only for a period within the current project period, not extending beyond it. Make the ending date of the supplement's first budget period coincide with the ending date of the budget period that is to be supplemented, regardless of the supplement's beginning date. If supplemental funds are being requested also for the future years of a currently funded grant, make the future years' budget periods coincide with the relevant budget periods of the currently funded grant.

NIH awarding components may not always be able to honor the requested start date of an applicant; accordingly, no commitments should be made or obligations created until confirmation of the actual start date by the awarding component.

All amounts requested must be in U.S. dollars.

Item 7a. Direct Costs Requested for Initial Budget Period. Enter the direct costs from form page 4.

Item 7b. Total Costs Requested for Initial Budget Period. Enter the sum of (1) the total direct costs on form page 4, and (2) the indirect costs for the initial budget period calculated on the checklist.

Item 8a. Direct Costs Requested for Entire Proposed Project Period. Enter the direct costs from form page 5.

Item 8b. Total Costs Requested for Entire Proposed Project Period. Enter the sum of (1) the total direct costs on form page 5, and (2) the indirect costs for the entire proposed project period calculated on the checklist.

Item 9. Performance Sites. Indicate where the work described in the Research Plan will be conducted. If there is more than one performance site, list all the sites, including V.A. facilities, and provide an explanation on the Resources and Environment page of the application. One of the sites indicated must be the applicant organization or be identified as off-site in accordance with the conditions of the appli-

cant organization's negotiated indirect cost agreement. This information must agree with the indirect cost information on the checklist of the application. State if a consortium/contractual arrangement is involved with one or more collaborating organizations for the relatively independent conduct of a portion of the work described in the Research Plan.

Item 10. Inventions and Patents (Competing Continuation Application Only). If no inventions were conceived or reduced to practice during the course of work under this project, check the box marked "NO." The remaining parts of Item 10 are then not applicable.

If any inventions were conceived or reduced to practice during the previous project period, check the box marked "YES" and list the titles of the inventions and the names of the inventors at the end of the progress report section of the Research Plan under a heading, "INVENTIONS." (This would ordinarily follow any listing of publications.) Also check the appropriate box to indicate whether this information has or has not been previously reported to the PHS or to the official responsible for patent matters in the applicant organization. The patent official must report these inventions promptly to the Extramural Inventions Office, NIH, Bethesda, MD 20892, Telephone: (301) 402-0850. This should be done prior to any publication or presentation of the invention at an open meeting, since failure to report at the appropriate time is a violation of 35 USC 202, and may result in loss of the rights of the applicant institution, inventor, and Federal Government in the invention. All foreign patent rights are immediately lost upon publication or other public disclosure unless a United States patent application is already on file. In addition, statutes preclude obtaining valid United States patent protection after one year from the date of a publication that discloses the invention.

Item 11. Applicant Organization. Name the **one** organization that will be legally and financially responsible for the conduct of activities supported by the award.

Item 12. Type of Organization. Check the appropriate box. If the applicant organization is public, specify whether it is Federal, State, or local. A Federal organization is a cabinet-level department or independent agency of the Executive Branch of the Federal Government or any component part of such a department or agency that may be assigned the responsibility for carrying out a grant-supported project. A Federal organization must submit with the completed application a certification of eligibility in accordance with the *PHS Grants Policy Statement*, Appendix V. A State organization is any agency or instrumentality of a State government of any of the United States or its territories. A local organization is any agency or instrumentality of a political subdivision of government below the State level.

A private nonprofit organization is an institution, corporation, or other legal entity no part of whose net earnings may lawfully inure to the benefit of any private shareholder or individual. A private nonprofit organization must submit proof of its nonprofit status if it has not previously done so. Acceptable proof to be submitted with the completed application may be: (a) a reference to the organization's listing in the most recent Internal Revenue Service cumulative list of tax exempt organizations; (b) a copy of a currently valid Internal Revenue Service tax exemption certificate; (c) a statement from a State taxing authority or State attorney general certifying that the organization is a nonprofit organization operating within the State, and that no part of its earnings may lawfully inure to the benefit of any private shareholder or individual; or (d) a certified copy of the certificate of incorporation or other document that clearly establishes the nonprofit status of the organization.

A forprofit organization is an institution, corporation, or other legal entity which is organized for the profit or benefit of its shareholders or other owners. A forprofit organization is considered to be a small business if it is independently owned and operated, if it is not dominant in the field of operation of the application, and if it employs fewer than 500 persons.

Item 13. Entity Identification Number.
Enter the number assigned to the applicant organization by the DHHS for payment and accounting purposes. If a number has not yet been assigned, enter the organization's Internal

Revenue Service employer identification number (nine digits). Also, enter the number of the Congressional District in the space provided.

Item 14. Biomedical Research Support Grant Credit.
This item is not applicable to Federal, foreign, or forprofit applicant organizations, nor to applications for Institutional National Research Service Awards and other training grants. For all other applications, identify the major component that is to receive credit towards eligibility for a Biomedical Research Support Grant should an award be made.

The component to receive credit must be the one responsible for the research and for administration of the award. For an application from a department or division that is shared by two or more schools of a university, designate the school having primary interest in the substance of the application.

Complete information is contained in the Biomedical Research Support Grant Information Statement and Administrative Guidelines. Copies of this statement may be obtained from the National Center for Research Resources, National Institutes of Health, Bethesda, MD 20892. Enter one of the following codes and identifications:

Academic Institutions	Nonacademic Institutions
Code Identification	**Code Identification**
01 School of Medicine	30 Hospital
03 School of Dentistry	52 Health Department
05 School of Osteopathy	60 Research Organization
07 School of Pharmacy	
09 School of Nursing	
11 School of Veterinary Medicine	
13 School of Public Health	
14 School of Optometry	
15 School of Allied Health	
16 College of Podiatric Medicine	
20 Other Academic	

Item 15. Administrative Official to be Notified if an Award is Made.
Provide a complete address for postal delivery. If the administrative official can receive electronic mail via BITNET or INTERNET, enter the appropriate electronic network address as the last line in this field.

Item 16. Official Signing for Applicant Organization.
Name an individual authorized

to act for the applicant organization and to assume the obligations imposed by the requirements and conditions for any grant, including the applicable Federal regulations. If the official signing for the applicant organization can receive electronic mail via BITNET or INTERNET, enter the appropriate electronic network address as the last line in this field.

Item 17. Principal Investigator/Program Director Assurance. An original signature in ink is required. "Per" signatures are not acceptable. Date of signature must be included.

Item 18. Certification and Acceptance. An original signature in ink is required. "Per" signatures are not acceptable. Date of signature must be included.

(Form Page 2)

Description. Follow instructions on form page 2.

Personnel. List *all* individuals, at the applicant organization or elsewhere, including the principal investigator, collaborating investigators, individuals in training, and support staff who will participate in the scientific execution of the project whether or not salaries are requested.

For every individual listed under Personnel, include all degrees, date of birth (format: Month-Day-Year), and Social Security Number (SSN). When requesting SSN, explain that provision is voluntary (See page 11). Also include the *Position Title* which is the position the individual occupies within his/her organization, e.g., assistant professor, staff researcher, predoctoral student, postdoctoral researcher, etc. Under *Role on the Project*, indicate how the individual will function with regard to the proposed project, for example, principal investigator, consultant, graduate research assistant, etc. Use an additional page in the same format as form page 2 if more space is necessary to list all personnel.

(Form Page 3)

RESEARCH GRANT TABLE OF CONTENTS

Number pages consecutively at the bottom of

each page throughout the application. Do not use suffixes such as 5a, 5b. Be sure to fill in the appropriate page numbers in the table of contents.

(Form Page 4)

DETAILED BUDGET PAGE FOR INITIAL BUDGET PERIOD.

List only the direct costs requested in this application. Do not include any items that are treated by the applicant organization as indirect costs according to a Federal rate negotiation agreement except for those indirect costs included in consortium/contractual costs. For a **Supplemental** application, do not use dollar amounts that were included in the budget of the parent application. Show only those items for which additional funds are requested, prorating the personnel costs and other appropriate parts of the detailed budget if the initial budget period of the supplemental application is less than 12 months. Budget periods of the supplement must coincide with the budget period of the parent grant. Each item must be clearly justified on form page 5.

Personnel

Name

Starting with the principal investigator, list the names and types of appointment of *all* personnel involved on the project during the initial budget period *who are employees* of the applicant organization regardless of whether a salary has been requested. Include all collaborating investigators, individuals in training, and support staff. The PHS does not recognize the co-principal investigator or co-investigator title as different from other collaborators.

Role on Project

Identify the role of each individual listed on the project. Describe their specific functions under Justification, on form page 5.

Type of Appointment/Months

List the number of months per year reflected in an individual's contractual appointment to the

16

applicant organization. **PHS staff assume that appointments at the applicant organization are full-time for each individual.** If an appointment is less than full-time (i.e., 1/2 time or 3/4), enter an asterisk (*) after the number of months and provide a full explanation under Justification, on form page 5. Individuals may have split appointments, for example, for an academic period and a summer period. For each appointment, identify and enter the number of months on separate lines. In cases where no contractual appointment exists with the applicant organization and salary is being requested, enter the number of months for that period.

Percent of Effort on Project

Percent of effort on project indicates the percent of each appointment at the applicant organization to be spent on this project.

Institutional Base Salary

Institutional base salary is defined as the annual compensation that the applicant organization pays for the individual's appointment, whether that individual's time is spent on research, teaching, patient care, or other activities. Base salary excludes any income that an individual may be permitted to earn outside of duties to the applicant organization. Base salary **may not** be increased as a result of replacing institutional salary funds with grant funds.

An applicant organization may choose to leave this column blank. However, PHS staff may require this information prior to award.

Dollar Amount Requested

Salary Requested

Enter the dollar amounts for each position for which funds are requested. The maximum salary that may be requested is calculated by multiplying the individual's base salary, defined above, by the percent of effort on this project. If a lesser amount is requested for any position, explain under Justification, on form page 5 (for example, endowed position, institutional sources, other support). Congress has imposed and may continue to impose salary caps. Applicants are

encouraged to contact their offices of sponsored programs or the *NIH Guide for Grants and Contracts* for current guidance. If an individual has used 2 or more lines to describe his/her type of appointment(s), and if a contractual appointment exists for only one of those periods, the requested monthly base salary for the other periods is calculated by dividing the institutional base salary by the number of months of the contractual appointment at the applicant organization.

Fringe Benefits

Fringe benefits may be requested in accordance with the *existing* rate agreement for each position provided such costs are treated consistently by the applicant organization as a direct cost to all sponsors.

Totals

Calculate the totals for each position and enter the **subtotals** in each column where indicated.

The applicant organization and its subcontractor(s) have the option of having specific salary and fringe benefit amounts for individuals omitted from copies of the application that are made available to non-Federal reviewers. If the applicant organization and its sub-contractors elect to exercise this option, use asterisks on the original and copies of the application to indicate those individuals for whom salaries and fringe benefits are being requested; the subtotals must still be shown. In addition, submit one copy of form page 4 of the application, completed in full with the asterisks replaced by the salaries and fringe benefits requested. This budget page will be reserved for PHS staff use only.

Consultant Costs

Whether or not costs are involved, provide the names and organizational affiliations of any consultants, other than those involved in consortium/contractual arrangements, who have agreed to serve in that capacity. Include consultant physicians in connection with patient care and persons who serve on external monitoring boards or advisory committees to the project. Briefly describe under Justification, form page 5, the services to be performed, including the number of days of anticipated consultation, the expected rate of compensation, travel, *per diem*, and other related costs.

Equipment

List separately each item of equipment with a unit acquisition cost of $500 or more. Justify the purchase under Justification, form page 5.

Supplies

Itemize supplies in separate categories such as glassware, chemicals, radioisotopes, etc. Categories in amounts less than $1,000 do not have to be itemized. If animals are involved, state the species, the number to be used, their unit purchase cost, their unit care cost, and the number of care days.

Travel

State, under Justification, form page 5, the purpose of any travel, giving the number of trips involved, the destinations, and the number of individuals for whom funds are requested.

Patient Care Costs

If inpatient and outpatient charges relevant to the research are requested, provide under Justification, form page 5, the names of the hospitals or clinics to be used and the amounts requested for each. State whether each hospital or clinic has a currently effective DHHS-negotiated patient care rate agreement, and if not, what basis is used for calculating charges. If an applicant does not have a DHHS-negotiated rate, a provisional rate can be approved by the PHS awarding component. Indicate in detail the basis for estimating costs in this category, including the number of patient days, estimated cost per day, and cost per test or treatment. Patient care costs do **not** include travel, lodging, subsistence, or donor/volunteer fees; request these costs in the **Other Expenses** category. Request consultant physician fees in the **Consultant Costs** category. Patient care costs will be provided to foreign organizations only in exceptional circumstances.

Alterations and Renovations

The costs of construction *per se* are not permissible charges. If the costs of essential alterations of facilities, including repairs, painting, removal or installation of partitions, shielding, or air conditioning are requested, itemize them by category and justify them fully under Justification, form page 5 . When applicable, indicate the square footage involved giving the basis for the costs, such as an architect's or contractor's detailed estimate. As required by the *PHS Grants Policy Statement,* line drawings of the proposed alterations should be submitted with the application. Costs for alterations and renovations are not allowed on grants made to foreign organizations.

Other Expenses

Itemize by category and unit cost such other expenses as publication costs, page charges, books, computer charges, rentals and leases, equipment maintenance, minor fee-for-service contracts, etc. Reimbursement is allowable for tuition remission in lieu of all or part of salary for student work on the project. State under Justification, form page 5, the percentage of tuition requested in proportion to the time devoted to the project. Reimbursement is allowable for donor/volunteer fees and for travel, lodging, and subsistence costs incurred by human subjects participating in the project, including travel of an escort, if required. This reimbursement is applicable to all classes of human subjects, including inpatients, outpatients, donors, and normal volunteers, regardless of employment status with the applicant organization. Detail such costs under Justification, form page 5.

Consortium/Contractual Costs

Each participating consortium/contractual organization must submit a separate detailed budget for the initial budget period and for the entire proposed project periods using copies of form pages 4 and 5.

Consortium arrangements may involve costs such as personnel, supplies, and any other allowable expenses, including indirect costs, for the relatively independent conduct of a portion of the work described in the Research Plan. Contractual arrangements for major support services, such as the laboratory testing of biological materials, clinical services, etc., are occasionally also of sufficient scope to warrant a similar categorical breakdown of costs. For either of the above arrangements, **enter both the total, direct, and indirect costs**. A separate budget page must be used for each subawardee.

List the indirect costs and provide the basis for the rate in the **Consortium/Contractual Costs** category for each supplementary budget page(s). Insert the page(s) after form page 5 numbering them sequentially. (Do not use 5a, 5b, 5c, etc.)

The **sum** of all consortium/contractual costs (direct costs and indirect costs), must be entered in the **Consortium/Contractual Costs** category of the applicant institution's budget.

(Form Page 5)

BUDGET FOR ENTIRE PROPOSED PROJECT PERIOD

Enter totals under each category for future years based on instructions for the initial budget period. If there are any significant increases or decreases in the future years, provide a justification.

Justification

Follow instructions on form page 5.

ADDITIONAL FORM PAGES

BIOGRAPHICAL SKETCH

This section should contain the biographical sketches of all *key personnel*, as well as all consultants and collaborators listed on form page 2. Key personnel include the principal investigator and any other individual who participates in the scientific development or execution of the project. Key personnel typically will include all individuals with doctoral or other professional degrees, but in some projects will include individuals at the masters or baccalaureate level provided they contribute in a substantive way to

the scientific development or execution of the project. References to publications must include titles and all authors. Do not exceed two pages for each biographical sketch.

OTHER SUPPORT

Other support is defined as any project specific funds or resources, whether Federal, non-Federal or institutional, available to the principal investigator/program director (and other key personnel named in the application) in direct support of their research endeavors through research or training grants, cooperative agreements, contracts, fellowships, gifts, prizes, and other means.

Information regarding active or pending sources of project specific support available to the principal investigator/program director (and other key personnel named in the application), whether related to this application or not, is an important part of the review and award process and must be included in this application. Please follow carefully the instructions and format on the *Other Support* page in providing this information.

RESOURCES AND ENVIRONMENT

Complete this section carefully. The information provided is critical to the review process.

C. SPECIFIC INSTRUCTIONS– Research Plan

Include sufficient, but concise information to facilitate an effective evaluation without having to review any previous application. Be specific and informative and avoid redundancies. Reviewers often consider brevity and clarity in the presentation to be indicative of a focused approach to a research objective and the ability to achieve the specific aims of the project.

Introduction (Revised or Supplemental Applications Only). All revised and supplemental applications must include an introduction. Do not exceed three pages for revised applications or one page for supplemental applications.

19

Revised Application. Acceptance of a revised application automatically withdraws the prior version. Summarize any substantial additions, deletions, and changes that have been made. The **Introduction** must include responses to criticisms in the previous summary statement. Highlight these changes within the text of the Research Plan by appropriate bracketing, indenting, or changing of typography. Do not underline or shade changes. Incorporate in the Progress Report/Preliminary Studies any work done since the prior version was submitted. **A revised application will be returned if it does not address criticisms in the previous summary statement and/or an introduction is not included and/or substantial revisions are not clearly apparent.**

Competitive Supplements. A competitive supplemental application may be submitted to request support for a significant expansion of a project's scope or research protocol. Competitive supplemental requests are **not** appropriate when the purpose is solely to restore, to the full IRG-recommended level, awards that were administratively reduced by the funding agency. A supplemental application will **not** be accepted until after the original application has been funded, and may not extend beyond the term of the current grant. The introduction to the supplemental application should provide an overall description of the nature of the supplement and how the supplement, or the lack thereof, will influence the specific aims, research design, and methods of the current grant. Any proposed changes in the allocation of funds within and among budget categories for the remainder of the project period of the current grant should be discussed under the budget justification. The body of the application should contain sufficient information from the original grant application to allow evaluation of the proposed supplement in relation to the goals of the original application.

If the supplemental application relates to a specific line of investigation, presented in the original application, that was not recommended for further consideration by the IRG, then the applicant must respond to the criticisms in the prior summary statement, and substantial revisions must be clearly evident and summarized in the introduction.

Research Plan. Organize Items 1-4, to answer these questions: (1) What do you intend to do? (2) Why is the work important? (3) What has already been done? (4) How are you going to do the work? **Do not exceed 25 pages for Items 1-4.** All tables and graphs must be included within the 25 page limit of Items 1-4. Full-sized glossy photographs of material such as electron micrographs or gels may be included in the Appendix; however, a copy of any such photograph must also be included within the Research Plan and within the page limitations (see Appendix for further instructions). **Twenty five pages is the absolute maximum and will be strictly enforced. Applications that exceed this limit, or that exceed the type size limitations (see page 10), will be returned without review.** You may use any page distribution within this overall limitation; however, the PHS recommends the following format and distribution:

1. **Specific Aims.** List the broad, long-term objectives and describe concisely and realistically what the specific research described in this application is intended to accomplish and any hypotheses to be tested. **One page is recommended.**

2. **Background and Significance.** Briefly sketch the background to the present proposal, critically evaluate existing knowledge, and specifically identify the gaps which the project is intended to fill. State concisely the importance of the research described in this application by relating the specific aims to the broad long-term objectives and to health relevance. **Two to three pages are recommended.**

3. **Progress Report/Preliminary Studies.** A progress report is required for **Competing Continuation and Supplemental** applications; for **New** applications, a report of the principal investigator/program director's preliminary studies is recommended.

    For **Competing Continuation** and **Supplemental** applications, give the beginning and ending dates for the period covered since the project was last reviewed competitively. List **all** personnel who have worked on the project during this period, their titles, birth dates, Social Security Numbers, dates of service, and percentages of their appointments devoted to the project. Summarize the previous application's specific aims and provide a succinct account of published and unpublished results indicating progress toward their achievement. Summarize the importance of the findings. Discuss any changes in the specific aims since the project was last reviewed competitively. List the titles and complete references to all publications, manuscripts **submitted or accepted** for publication, patents, invention reports, and other printed materials that have resulted from the project since it was last reviewed competitively. **Note that this list is excluded from the 25 page limit.** Submit five collated sets of **no more than 10** such items as an Appendix.

New applications may use this section to provide an account of the principal investigator/program director's preliminary studies pertinent to the application and/or any other information that will help to establish the experience and competence of the investigator to pursue the proposed project. The titles and complete references to appropriate publications and manuscripts **submitted or accepted** for publication may be listed, and five collated sets of **no more than 10** such items of background material may be submitted in the Appendix. **Six to eight pages are recommended for the narrative portion of the Progress Report/Preliminary Studies, excluding the list of materials resulting from the project since it was last reviewed competitively.**

4. **Research Design and Methods.** Describe the research design and the procedures to be used to accomplish the specific aims of the project. Include the means by which the data will be collected, analyzed, and interpreted. Describe any new methodology and its advantage over existing methodologies. Discuss the potential difficulties and limitations of the proposed procedures and alternative approaches to achieve the aims. Provide a tentative sequence or timetable for the investigation. Point out any procedures, situations, or materials that may be hazardous to personnel and the precautions to be exercised. **Although no specific number of pages is recommended for this section of the application, the total for Items 1-4 may not exceed 25 pages, including all tables and figures.**

Gender and Minority Inclusion: Applications for grants and cooperative agreements that involve human subjects are required to include minorities and both genders in study populations so that research findings can be of benefit to all persons at risk of the disease, disorder, or condition under study; special emphasis should be placed on the need for inclusion of minorities and women in studies of diseases, disorders, and conditions which disproportionately affect them. This policy applies to **all** research involving human subjects and human materials, and applies to males and females of all ages. If one gender and/or minorities are excluded or are inadequately represented in this research, particularly in proposed population-based studies, a clear compelling rationale for exclusion or inadequate representation should be provided. The composition of the proposed study population must be described in terms of gender and racial/ethnic group, together with a rationale for its choice. In addition, gender and racial/ethnic issues should be addressed in developing a research design and sample size appropriate for the scientific objectives of the study.

Assess carefully the feasibility of including the broadest possible representation of minority groups. However, NIH and ADAMHA recognize that it may not be feasible or appropriate in all research projects to include representation of the full array of United States racial/ethnic minority populations (i.e., American Indians or Alaskan Natives, Asians or Pacific Islanders, Blacks, Hispanics). Provide the rationale for studies on single minority population groups.

Applications for support of research involving human subjects must employ a study design with gender and/or minority representation (by age distribution, risk factors, incidence/prevalence, etc.) appropriate to the scientific objectives of the research. It is not an automatic requirement for the study design to provide statistical power to answer the questions posed for men and women and racial/ethnic groups separately; however, whenever there are scientific reasons to anticipate differences between men and women, and racial/ethnic groups, with regard to the hypothesis under investigation, applicants should include an evaluation of these gender and minority group differences in the proposed study. If adequate inclusion of one gender and/or minorities is impossible or inappropriate with respect to the purpose of the research because of the health of the subjects, or other reasons, or if in the only study population available, there is a disproportionate representation of one gender or minority/majority group, the rationale for the study population must be well explained and justified.

5. **Human Subjects.** If you have marked Item 4a on the Face Page "YES" and designated exemptions from the human subjects regulations, **provide sufficient information to allow a determination that the designated exemptions are appropriate.** Research that is exempt from coverage under the regulations is discussed under Human Subjects in the Discussion of Assurance and Certification Requirements, page 25. **Although a grant application is exempt from these regulations, it must, nevertheless, address the issues of gender/race/ethnic composition of the subject population as instructed.**

If you have marked Item 4a on the Face Page of the application "YES," and designated no exemptions from the regulations, the following six points **must be addressed**. In addition, when research involving human subjects will take place at collaborating site(s) or other performance site(s), provide this information before the six points are discussed. **Although no specific page limitation applies to this section of the application, be succinct.**

(1) Provide a detailed description of the proposed involvement of human subjects in the work previously outlined in the Research Design and Methods section. Describe the characteristics of the subject population, including their anticipated number, age range, and health status. Summarize the gender and racial/ethnic composition of the subject population. Identify the criteria for inclusion or exclusion of any subpopulation. **If one gender and/or minorities are not included in a given study, provide a clear rationale for their exclusion.** Explain the rationale for the involvement of special classes of subjects, if any, such as fetuses, pregnant women, children, human in vitro fertilization, prisoners or other institutionalized individuals, or others who are likely to be vulnerable.

(2) Identify the sources of research material obtained from individually identifiable **living** human subjects in the form of specimens, records, or data. Indicate whether the material or data will be obtained specifically for research purposes or whether use will be made of existing specimens, records, or data.

(3) Describe plans for the recruitment of subjects and the consent procedures to be followed, including the circumstances under which consent will be sought and obtained, who will seek it, the nature of the information to be provided to prospective subjects, and the method of documenting consent. State if the Institutional Review Board (IRB) has authorized a modification or waiver of the elements of consent or the requirement for documentation of consent. The informed consent form, which must have IRB approval, should be submitted to the PHS only on request.

(4) Describe any potential risks (physical, psychological, social, legal, or other) and assess their likelihood and seriousness. Where appropriate, describe alternative treatments and procedures that might be advantageous to the subjects.

(5) Describe the procedures for protecting against or minimizing any potential risks, including risks to confidentiality, and assess their likely effectiveness. Where appropriate, discuss provisions for ensuring neces-

sary medical or professional intervention in the event of adverse effects to the subjects. Also, where appropriate, describe the provisions for monitoring the data collected to ensure the safety of subjects.

(6) Discuss why the risks to subjects are reasonable in relation to the anticipated benefits to subjects and in relation to the importance of the knowledge that may reasonably be expected to result.

If a test article (investigational new drug, device, or biologic) is involved, name the test article and state whether the 30-day interval between submission of applicant certification to the Food and Drug Administration and its response has elapsed or has been waived and/or whether use of the test article has been withheld or restricted by the Food and Drug Administration.

6. **Vertebrate Animals.** If you have marked Item 5a on the Face Page of the application "YES," the following five points **must be addressed**. In addition, when research involving vertebrate animals will take place at collaborating site(s) or other performance site(s), provide this information before the five points are discussed.

Although no specific page limitation applies to this section of the application, be succinct.

(1) Provide a detailed description of the proposed use of the animals in the work previously outlined in the research design and methods section. Identify the species, strains, ages, sex, and numbers of animals to be used in the proposed work.

(2) Justify the use of animals, the choice of species, and the numbers used. If animals are in short supply, costly, or to be used in large numbers, provide an additional rationale for their selection and numbers.

(3) Provide information on the veterinary care of the animals involved.

(4) Describe the procedures for ensuring

that discomfort, distress, pain, and injury will be limited to that which is unavoidable in the conduct of scientifically sound research. Describe the use of analgesic, anesthetic, and tranquilizing drugs and/or comfortable restraining devices, where appropriate, to minimize discomfort, distress, pain, and injury.

(5) Describe any method of euthanasia to be used and the reasons for its selection. State whether this method is consistent with the recommendations of the Panel on Euthanasia of the American Veterinary Medical Association. If **not,** present a justification for not following the recommendations.

7. **Consultants/Collaborators.** List all consultants and collaborators involved with this project, whether or not salaries are requested. Attach an appropriate letter from each individual confirming his or her role on the project. **Do not place these letters in the Appendix.** Also include Biographical Sketch pages for each consultant and collaborator and place them with those of the other participants on the project.

8. **Consortium/Contractual Arrangements.** Provide a detailed explanation of the programmatic, fiscal, and administrative arrangements made between the applicant organization and the collaborating organizations. Provide a statement that the applicant organization and the collaborating organizations have established or are prepared to establish written interorganizational agreements that will ensure compliance with all pertinent Federal regulations and policies. Attach confirming letters countersigned by an authorized official of the collaborating institutions and principal investigator or copies of written agreements.

If consortium/contractual activities represent a significant portion of the overall project, explain why the applicant organization, rather than the ultimate performer of the activities, should be the grantee. The major purpose of this requirement is to ensure that the applicant organization intends to perform a substantive role in the conduct of the project, as prescribed by PHS grants policy.

23

9. **Literature Cited.** Do not scatter literature citations throughout the text. List them at the end of the Research Plan. The list may include, but may not replace, the list of publications in the Progress Report required for **Competing Continuation** and **Supplemental** applications. Each literature citation **must include** the title, names of all authors, book or journal, volume number, page numbers, and year of publication. Make every attempt to be judicious in compiling a relevant and current list of literature citations; it need not be exhaustive. **Do not exceed six pages**.

D. SPECIFIC INSTRUCTIONS– Appendix

Appendix

An application may be returned if the appendix fails to observe the limitations on content. These limitations may not apply to the specialized grant applications listed in the section entitled Types of Applications and Required Forms (page 5). Request and follow the additional instructions for those applications.

Appendix material may include questionnaires, photographs (see below), or other materials that do not copy well. For **Competing Continuation** and **Supplemental** applications, submit five collated sets of **no more than 10** publications, manuscripts **submitted or accepted** for publication, patents, invention reports, and other printed materials that have resulted from the project since it was last reviewed competitively. Five collated sets of similar printed background material documenting preliminary studies may also be appended to new applications. Individual manuscripts within the appendix should be stapled, although the rest of the application should not be stapled (see page 7).

Full-sized glossy photographs of material such as electron micrographs, gels, etc. may be included in the Appendix, **provided a photocopy** (which could be reduced in size from the glossy photograph in the Appendix) **is included within the 25 page limit of Sections 1-4 of the Research Plan.** All other graphs, diagrams, tables, and charts must be included within the 25 page limit of Sections 1-4 in the Research Plan. The Appendix is **not** to be used to circumvent the page limitations in the Research Plan. The Appendix will **not** be duplicated with the rest of the application and only selected members of IRG will receive this material.

Include five collated sets of all appendix material in the application package. Appendix material should be grouped **after** all copies of the application. Do not mail this material separately. Identify each of the sets with the name of the principal investigator/program director and the project title.

E. SPECIFIC INSTRUCTIONS– Checklist (Complete both pages)

1. Assurances and Certifications

Each application to the PHS requires that the following assurances and certifications be provided, as appropriate:

Human Subjects
Vertebrate Animals
Inventions and Patents
Debarment and Suspension
Drug-Free Workplace
Lobbying
Delinquent Federal Debt
Misconduct in Science
Civil Rights
Handicapped Individuals
Sex Discrimination
Age Discrimination

The following paragraphs refer to each required assurance and give specific instructions for completing the **Checklist**. In addition, specific information related to human subjects, inclusion of both genders and minorities in study populations, and vertebrate animals is required in the research plan of the application itself.

The assurances/certifications described below are made by checking the appropriate boxes on the **Face Page** as well as those on the **Checklist** portion of the application. They are verified by the signature of the **Official Signing For Applicant Organization** on the **Face Page** of the application.

24

a. Human Subjects (Complete Item 4 on the Face Page)

The DHHS regulations for the protection of human subjects provide a systematic means, based on established, internationally recognized ethical principles, to safeguard the rights and welfare of individuals who participate as subjects in research activities supported or conducted by the DHHS. The regulations require that applicant organizations establish and maintain appropriate policies and procedures for the protection of human subjects. These regulations, 45 CFR 46, Protection of Human Subjects, are available from the Office for Protection from Research Risks, National Institutes of Health, Bethesda, MD 20892, Telephone: (301) 496-7041.

The regulations stipulate that an applicant organization, whether domestic or foreign, bears responsibility for safeguarding the rights and welfare of human subjects in DHHS-supported research activities. The regulations define "human subject" as "a living individual about whom an investigator (whether professional or student) conducting research obtains (1) data through intervention or interaction with the individual or (2) identifiable private information." The regulations extend to the use of human organs, tissues, and body fluids from individually identifiable human subjects as well as to graphic, written, or recorded information derived from individually identifiable human subjects. The use of autopsy materials is governed by applicable state and local law and is not directly regulated by 45 CFR 46.

Research involving human subjects may be classified as non-exempt or exempt (see next paragraph). An applicant organization proposing to do non-exempt research must file an Assurance of Compliance with the Office for Protection from Research Risks (OPRR). As part of this Assurance, which commits the applicant organization to comply with the DHHS regulations, the applicant organization must appoint an Institutional Review Board (IRB), which is required to review and approve all nonexempt research activities involving human subjects.

Research which is exempt from coverage by the regulations are activities in which the only involvement of human subjects will be in one or more of the following six categories:

(1) Research conducted in established or commonly accepted educational settings, involving normal educational practices, such as (a) research on regular and special education instructional strategies, or (b) research on the effectiveness of or the comparison among instructional techniques, curricula, or classroom management methods.

(2) Research involving the use of educational tests (cognitive, diagnostic, aptitude, achievement), survey procedures, interview procedures or observation of public behavior, unless: (a) information obtained is recorded in such a manner that human subjects can be identified, directly or through identifiers linked to the subjects; and (b) any disclosure of the human subjects' responses outside the research could reasonably place the subjects at risk of criminal or civil liability or be damaging to the subjects' financial standing, employability, or reputation.

(3) Research involving the use of educational tests (cognitive, diagnostic, aptitude, achievement), survey procedures, interview procedures, or observation of public behavior that is not exempt under paragraph(2) (b) of this section, if: (a) the human subjects are elected or appointed public officials or candidates for public office; or (b) federal statute(s) require(s) without exception that the confidentiality of the personally identifiable information will be maintained throughout the research and thereafter.

(4) Research, involving the collection or study of existing data, documents, records, pathological specimens, or diagnostic specimens, if these sources are publicly available or if the information is recorded by the investigator in such a manner that subjects cannot be identified, directly or through identifiers linked to the subjects.

(5) Research and demonstration projects which are conducted by or subject to the approval of department or agency heads,

and which are designed to study, evaluate, or otherwise examine: (a) public benefit or service programs; (b) procedures for obtaining benefits or services under those programs; (c) possible changes in or alternatives to those programs or procedures; or (d) possible changes in methods or levels of payment for benefits or services under those programs.

(6)　Taste and food quality evaluation and consumer acceptance studies, (a) if wholesome foods without additives are consumed or (b) if a food is consumed that contains a food ingredient at or below the level and for a use found to be safe, or agricultural chemical or environmental contaminant at or below the level found to be safe, by the Food and Drug Administration or approved by the Environmental Protection Agency or the Food Safety and Inspection Service of the U.S. Department of Agriculture.

Investigators who conduct research involving fetuses, pregnant women, children, human *in vitro* fertilization, or prisoners must follow the provisions of the regulations in Subparts B, C, and D of 45 CFR 46, which describe the additional protections required for these subjects.

No DHHS award for non-exempt research involving human subjects will be made to an applicant organization unless that organization is operating in accord with an approved Assurance of Compliance and provides certification that the IRB has reviewed and approved the proposed activity in accordance with the DHHS regulations. Copies of the approved Assurance of Compliance are available to every researcher at the applicant organization. No award to an individual will be made unless that individual is affiliated with an organization that accepts responsibility for compliance with the DHHS regulations and has filed the necessary Assurance with OPRR. Foreign applicant organizations must also comply with the provisions of the regulations.

Research investigators are entrusted with an essential role in assuring the adequate protection of human subjects. In activities they conduct or which are conducted under their direction,

they have a direct and continuing responsibility to safeguard the rights and the welfare of the individuals who are or may become subjects of the research. Investigators must comply with the DHHS regulations, with the applicant organization's Assurance of Compliance, and with the requirements and determinations of the IRB concerning the conduct of the research. Investigators must avoid unnecessary risks to subjects by using procedures which are consistent with sound research design and acceptable medical practice. Whenever appropriate, investigators should use procedures already being performed on the subjects for diagnostic or treatment purposes. Risks to subjects must be reasonable in relation to anticipated benefits, if any, to subjects, and to the importance of the knowledge that may reasonably be expected to result. Investigators must obtain the legally effective informed consent of each subject or of the subject's legally authorized representative before involving the subject in the research, to the extent required by and in accordance with 45 CFR 46, or as required by applicable Federal, State, or local law. The consent form must be approved by the IRB.

b.　Vertebrate Animals (Complete Item 5 on the Face Page)

The Public Health Service (PHS) Policy on Humane Care and Use of Laboratory Animals requires that applicant organizations establish and maintain appropriate policies and procedures to ensure the humane care and use of live vertebrate animals involved in research activities supported by the PHS. This policy implements and supplements the *U.S. Government Principles for the Utilization and Care of Vertebrate Animals Used in Testing, Research, and Training* and requires that institutions use the *Guide for the Care and Use of Laboratory Animals* as a basis for developing and implementing an institutional animal care and use program. This policy does not affect applicable State or local laws or regulations which impose more stringent standards for the care and use of laboratory animals. All institutions are required to comply, as applicable, with the Animal Welfare Act as amended (7 USC 2131 et seq.), and other Federal statutes and regulations relating to animals. These documents are available from the Office for Protection from Research Risks, National Institutes of Health, Bethesda, MD 20892, Telephone: (301) 496-7163.

The PHS policy stipulates that an applicant organization, whether domestic or foreign, bears responsibility for the humane care and use of animals in PHS-supported research activities. The PHS policy defines "animal" as "any live, vertebrate animal used or intended for use in research, research training, experimentation or biological testing or for related purposes." An applicant organization proposing to use vertebrate animals in PHS-supported activities must file an Animal Welfare Assurance with the OPRR. As part of this Assurance, which commits the applicant organization to comply with the PHS policy, the applicant organization must appoint an Institutional Animal Care and Use Committee (IACUC) which is required to review and approve those sections of applications for PHS support that involve vertebrate animals.

No PHS award for research involving vertebrate animals will be made to an applicant organization unless that organization is operating in accordance with an approved Animal Welfare Assurance and provides verification that the IACUC has reviewed and approved the proposed activity in accordance with the PHS policy. Applications may be referred by the PHS back to the IACUC for further review in the case of apparent or potential violations of the PHS policy. Copies of the approved Animal Welfare Assurance are available to every researcher at the applicant organization. No award to an individual will be made unless that individual is affiliated with an organization that accepts responsibility for compliance with the PHS policy and has filed the necessary Assurance with OPRR. Foreign applicant organizations applying for PHS awards for activities involving vertebrate animals are required to comply with PHS policy or provide evidence that acceptable standards for the humane care and use of animals will be met.

Research investigators are entrusted with an essential role in assuring the humane care and use of animals. In activities they conduct or which are conducted under their direction, they have a direct and continuing responsibility to see that animals are adequately cared for and used.

Investigators must comply with the PHS policy, with the applicant organization's Animal Welfare Assurance, and with the requirements and determinations of the IACUC concerning the conduct of the research. Investigators must ensure that discomfort, distress, pain, and injury to the animals are avoided or minimized, consistent with sound research design; that no more animals are used than are necessary to reach sound scientific conclusions; and that, when appropriate, animals are painlessly sacrificed in accordance with methods of euthanasia approved by the Panel on Euthanasia of the American Veterinary Medical Association.

c. Inventions and Patents (Competing Continuation Application Only - Complete Item 10 on the Face Page)

d. Debarment and Suspension

Executive Order 12549, "Debarment and Suspension," calls for development of a **Governmentwide** debarment and suspension system for nonprocurement transactions with Federal agencies. "Nonprocurement" transactions include grants, cooperative agreements, and fellowships. DHHS regulations implementing Executive Order 12549 are provided in 45 CFR 76, "Governmentwide Debarment and Suspension (Nonprocurement) and Governmentwide Requirements for Drug-Free Workplace (Grants)." Accordingly, before a grant award can be made, the applicant organization must make the following certification (Appendix A of the DHHS regulations):

"(1) The prospective primary participant certifies to the best of its knowledge and belief, that it and its principals (including research personnel):

"(a) Are not presently debarred, suspended, proposed for debarment, declared ineligible, or voluntarily excluded from covered transactions by any Federal department or agency;

"(b) Have not within a three-year period preceding this proposal been convicted of or had a civil judgment rendered against them for commission of fraud or a criminal offense in connection with obtaining, attempting to obtain, or performing a public (Federal, State, or local) transaction or contract under a public transaction; violation of Federal or State antitrust statutes or commission of embezzlement, theft, forgery, bribery, falsification or destruction of records, making false statements, or receiving stolen property;

"(c) Are not presently indicted for or otherwise criminally or civilly charged by a governmental entity (Federal, State, or local) with commission of any of the offenses enumerated in paragraph (1)(b) of this certification; and

"(d) Have not within a three-year period preceding this application/proposal had one or more public transactions (Federal, State, or local) terminated for cause or default.

"(2) Where the prospective primary participant is unable to certify to any of the statements in this certification, such prospective participant shall attach an explanation to this proposal."

Grantees are required to obtain a similar certification from most subawardees (called "lower tier participants"). See 45 CFR 76, Appendices A and B.

e. Drug-Free Workplace (Applicable only to new or revised applications being submitted to the PHS for the first proposed project period [Type 1])

The Drug-Free Workplace Act of 1988 (Public Law 100-690, Title V, Subtitle D) requires that all grantees receiving grants from any Federal agency certify to that agency that they will maintain a drug-free workplace. DHHS regulations implementing the Act are provided in 45 CFR 76, "Governmentwide Debarment and Suspension (Nonprocurement) and Governmentwide Requirements for Drug-Free Workplace (Grants)." Accordingly, before a grant award can be made, the applicant organization must make the certification set forth below (Appendix C of the DHHS regulations). The certification is a material representation of fact upon which reliance will be placed by the PHS awarding component. False certification or violation of the certification shall be grounds for suspension of payments, suspension or termination of grants, or **Governmentwide** suspension or debarment.

The applicant organization certifies "that it will continue to provide a drug-free workplace by:

"(a) Publishing a statement notifying employees that the unlawful manufacture, distribution, dispensing, possession or use of a controlled substance is prohibited in the grantee's workplace and specifying the actions that will be taken against employees for violation of such prohibition;

"(b) Establishing an ongoing drug-free awareness program to inform employees about:

"(1) The dangers of drug abuse in the workplace;

"(2) The grantee's policy of maintaining a drug-free workplace;

"(3) Any available drug counseling, rehabilitation, and employee assistance programs; and

"(4) The penalties that may be imposed upon employees for drug abuse violations occurring in the workplace;

"(c) Making it a requirement that each employee to be engaged in the performance of the grant be given a copy of the statement required by paragraph (a);

"(d) Notifying the employee in the statement required by paragraph (a) that, as a condition of employment under the grant, the employee will:

"(1) Abide by the terms of the statement; and

"(2) Notify the employer in writing of his or her conviction for a violation of a

28

criminal drug statute occurring in the workplace no later than five calendar days after such conviction;

"(e) Notifying the agency in writing within 10 calendar days after receiving notice under subparagraph (d)(2) from an employee or otherwise receiving actual notice of such conviction. Employers of convicted employees must provide notice, including position title, to every grant officer or other designee on whose grant activity the convicted employee was working, unless the Federal agency has designated a central point for the receipt of such notices. Notice shall include the identification number(s) of each affected grant;

"(f) Taking one of the following actions, within 30 calendar days of receiving notice under subparagraph (d)(2), with respect to any employee who is so convicted:

"(1) Taking appropriate personnel action against such an employee, up to and including termination, consistent with the requirements of the Rehabilitation Act of 1973, as amended; or

"(2) Requiring such employee to participate satisfactorily in a drug abuse assistance or rehabilitation program approved for such purposes by a Federal, State, or local health, law enforcement, or other appropriate agency;

"(g) Making a good faith effort to continue to maintain a drug-free workplace through implementation of paragraphs (a), (b), (c), (d), (e), and (f)."

For purposes of paragraph (e) regarding agency notification of criminal drug convictions, the DHHS has designated the following central point for receipt of such notices:

Division of Grants Management and Oversight
Office of Management and Acquisition
Department of Health and Human Services
Room 517-D
200 Independence Avenue, S.W.
Washington, DC 20201

f. Lobbying

Title 31, United States Code, Section 1352, entitled "Limitation on Use of Appropriated Funds to Influence Certain Federal Contracting and Financial Transactions," generally prohibits recipients of Federal grants and cooperative agreements from using Federal (appropriated) funds for lobbying the Executive or Legislative Branches of the Federal Government in connection with a **specific** grant or cooperative agreement. Section 1352 also requires that each person who requests or receives a Federal grant or cooperative agreement must disclose lobbying undertaken with non-Federal (nonappropriated) funds. These requirements apply to grants and cooperative agreements **exceeding** $100,000 in total costs.

The complete Certification Regarding Lobbying is provided below. "The undersigned (authorized official signing for the applicant organization) certifies, to the best of his or her knowledge and belief, that:

"(1) No Federal appropriated funds have been paid or will be paid, by or on behalf of the undersigned, to any person for influencing or attempting to influence an officer or employee of any agency, a Member of Congress, an officer or employee of Congress, or an employee of a Member of Congress in connection with the awarding of any Federal contract, the making of any Federal grant, the making of any Federal loan, the entering into of any cooperative agreement, and the extension, continuation, renewal, amendment, or modification of any Federal contract, grant, loan, or cooperative agreement.

"(2) If any funds other than Federally appropriated funds have been paid or will be paid to any person for influencing or attempting to influence an officer or employee of any agency, a Member of Congress, an officer or employee of Congress, or an employee of a Member of Congress in connection with this Federal contract, grant, loan, or cooperative agreement, the undersigned shall complete and submit Standard Form-LLL, "Disclosure of Lobbying Activities," in accordance with its instructions.

29

"(3) The undersigned shall require that the language of this certification be included in the award documents for all subawards at all tiers (including subcontracts, subgrants, and contracts under grants, loans and cooperative agreements) and that all subrecipients shall certify and disclose accordingly.

"This certification is a material representation of fact upon which reliance was placed when this transaction was made or entered into. Submission of this certification is a prerequisite for making or entering into this transaction imposed by Section 1352, U.S. Code. Any person who fails to file the required certification shall be subject to a civil penalty of not less than $10,000 and not more than $100,000 for each such failure."

Standard Form-LLL, "Disclosure of Lobbying Activities," its instructions, and continuation sheet are available from the Office of Grants Inquiries, Division of Research Grants, National Institutes of Health, Bethesda, MD 20892, Telephone: (301) 496-7441. If required, complete and sign the form and attach it to the application behind the second page of the Checklist.

g. Delinquent Federal Debt

A major goal of Office of Management and Budget Circular No. A-129, "Managing Federal Credit Programs," is the collection of delinquent Federal debt. Accordingly, before a grant award can be made, the applicant organization must certify that it is **not** delinquent on the repayment of any Federal debt. The certification applies to the applicant organization, **not** to the person signing the application as the authorized representative **nor** to the principal investigator/program director.

Examples of Federal debt include delinquent taxes, audit disallowances, guaranteed or direct student loans, FHA loans, business loans, and other miscellaneous administrative debts. For purposes of this certification, the following definitions of "delinquency" apply:

- For **direct loans and fellowships** (whether awarded directly to the applicant by the Federal Government or by an institution using

Federal funds), a debt more than 31 days past due on a scheduled payment. (Definition **excludes** "service" payback under a National Research Service Award.)

- For **guaranteed and insured loans**, recipients of a loan guaranteed by the Federal Government that the Federal Government has repurchased from a lender because the borrower breached the loan agreement and is in default.

- For **grants**, organizations in receipt of "Notice of Grants Cost Disallowance" which have not repaid the disallowed amount or which have not resolved the disallowance. (Definition **excludes** cost disallowances in an "appeal" status.)

Where the applicant discloses delinquency on debt to the Federal Government, the PHS shall (1) take such information into account when determining whether the prospective grantee organization is responsible with respect to that grant, and (2) consider not making the grant until payment is made or satisfactory arrangements are made with the agency to whom the debt is owed. Therefore, it may be necessary for the PHS to contact the applicant before a grant can be made to confirm the status of the debt and ascertain the payment arrangements for its liquidation. Applicants who fail to liquidate indebtedness to the Federal Government in a business-like manner place themselves at risk of not receiving financial assistance from the PHS.

h. Misconduct in Science

Scientific misconduct is defined by PHS as fabrication, falsification, plagiarism, or other practices that seriously deviate from those that are commonly accepted within the scientific community for proposing, conducting, or reporting research. It does not include honest error or honest differences in interpretations or judgments of data. It also does not include material failure to comply with Federal requirements affecting specific aspects of the conduct of research, e.g., the protection of human subjects and the welfare of laboratory animals. Validation of these requirements is handled by other PHS offices.

30

Each institution which receives or applies for a research, research training, or research related grant or cooperative agreement under the Public Health Service Act must submit an annual assurance. This certifies that the institution has established administrative policies as required by the "Final Rule Regarding Responsibilities of Awardee and Applicant Institutions for Dealing with and Reporting Possible Misconduct in Science" (42 CFR Part 50, Subpart A), and that it will comply with those policies and the requirements of the Final Rule. These regulations are available from the Office of Scientific Integrity, National Institutes of Health, Bethesda, MD 20892, Telephone: (301)496-2624.

The signature of the official signing for the applicant organization on the **Face Page** of the application serves as certification that the institution has submitted an assurance that:

(a) The organization has established—and will comply with—policies and procedures, incorporating the provisions set forth in 42 CFR Part 50, Subpart A;

(b) The organization will comply with the requirements of the PHS regulations on responsibilities of awardee and applicant institutions for dealing with and reporting possible misconduct in science (42 CFR Part 50, Subpart A); and

(c) The organization will provide its policies and procedures to the PHS upon request.

The date of the Initial Assurance or latest Annual Report submission to the Office of Scientific Integrity should be indicated in Item h of the Checklist.

i. Civil Rights

Before a grant award can be made, a domestic applicant organization must certify that it has filed with the DHHS Office for Civil Rights an Assurance of Compliance (Form HHS 441) with Title VI of the Civil Rights Act of 1964 (42 USC 2000d). This provides that no person in the United States shall, on the grounds of race, color, or national origin, be excluded from participation in, be denied the benefits of, or be other-

wise subjected to discrimination under any program or activity receiving Federal financial assistance. The pertinent DHHS implementing regulations are found in 45 CFR 80.

j. Handicapped Individuals

Before a grant award can be made, a domestic applicant organization must certify that it has filed with the DHHS Office for Civil Rights an Assurance of Compliance (Form HHS 641) with Section 504 of the Rehabilitation Act of 1973, as amended (29 USC 794). This provides that no handicapped individual in the United States shall, solely by reason of the handicap, be excluded from participation in, be denied the benefits of, or be subjected to discrimination under any program or activity receiving Federal financial assistance. The pertinent DHHS implementing regulations are found in 45 CFR 84.

k. Sex Discrimination

Before a grant award can be made, a domestic, applicant educational organization (or any domestic non-educational organization which has applied for training grant support) must certify that it has filed with the DHHS Office for Civil Rights an Assurance of Compliance (Form HHS 639-A) with Section 901 of Title IX of the Education Amendments of 1972 (20 USC 1681) as amended. This provides that no person in the United States shall, on the basis of sex, be excluded from participation in, be denied the benefits of, or be subjected to discrimination under any education program or activity receiving Federal financial assistance. The pertinent DHHS implementing regulations are found in 45 CFR 86.

l. Age Discrimination

Before a grant award can be made, a domestic applicant organization must certify that it has filed with the DHHS Office for Civil Rights an Assurance of Compliance (Form HHS 680) with the Age Discrimination Act of 1975. The Act prohibits unreasonable discrimination on the basis of age in any program or activity receiving Federal financial assistance. Specifically, no person in the United States shall, on the basis of age, be denied the benefits of, be excluded from participation in, or be subjected to discrimination under any program or activity receiving Federal financial assistance. The pertinent DHHS implementing regulations are found in 45 CFR 91.

The Assurance of Compliance Forms HHS 441, 641, 639-A, and 680 are available from the Office of Grants Inquiries, Division of Research Grants, National Institutes of Health, Bethesda, MD 20892.

2. Program Income

Program income is gross income earned by a research grant recipient from activities part or all of which are borne as a direct cost by the grant. The *PHS Grants Policy Statement* contains a detailed explanation of program income, the ways in which it may be generated and accounted for, and the various options for its use and disposition.

Examples of program income include:

- Fees earned from services performed under the grant, such as those resulting from laboratory drug testing;

- Rental or usage fees, such as those earned from fees charged for use of computer equipment purchased with grant funds;

- Third party patient reimbursement for hospital or other medical services, such as insurance payments for patients where such reimbursement occurs because of the grant-supported activity;

- Funds generated by the sale of commodities, such as tissue cultures, cell lines, or research animals; and

- Patent or copyright royalties.

If no program income is anticipated during the period(s) for which grant support is requested, check the box marked "NO" on page 2 of the Checklist. No other action is necessary.

If the response to this item is "YES," check the appropriate box and follow the prescribed format to reflect, by budget period, the amount and source(s) of anticipated program income. If the application is funded, the Notice of Grant Award will provide specific instructions regarding the use of such income. (See *PHS Grants Policy Statement* for PHS policy on the treatment of program income earned under research grants.)

3. Indirect Costs - see Checklist - self-explanatory.

F. PERSONAL DATA FORM - self-explanatory.

V. ADDITIONAL INFORMATION

A. INTERACTIONS BETWEEN THE PRINCIPAL INVESTIGATOR/PROGRAM DIRECTOR AND THE PHS AFTER SUBMISSION OF AN APPLICATION

The PHS automatically informs both the principal investigator/program director and the administrative official of the applicant organization about the acceptance of an application and its assignment to an IRG and Institute. As soon as possible after each IRG meeting, the principal investigator/program director is automatically sent the priority score and percentile rank. In addition, most components of the PHS automatically send the principal investigator/program director a summary statement of the IRG's findings and recommendations with the priority score and percentile rank displayed. If the council or board recommends an action other than that recommended by the IRG, the PHS will send a letter to the principal investigator/program director indicating the action and its rationale. Subsequent decisions concerning the funding of applications will take into account elements such as the relevance of the goals of the proposed research to the missions of the awarding component, program balance, overlapping support from other sources, and the availability of funds. The PHS will notify the principal investigator/program director and the applicant organization of the final disposition of the application.

A principal investigator/program director can interact with the PHS several times throughout the process. At the time of submission, an applicant may include a cover letter with the application requesting up to three IRGs and/or an awarding component to which the application could be assigned. These suggestions will be taken into consideration at the time of assignment, although the final determination will be made by the PHS. If an application is assigned to an Institute or IRG that the applicant thinks inappropriate, the applicant should immediately contact the Referral Office at (301) 496-7447 to discuss the possibility of reassignment. Telephone requests should be followed by written requests to the Referral Office. These requests will be carefully considered, but, again, the final determination will be made by PHS.

Once the most appropriate assignment has been made, any questions or concerns about the review of the application should be addressed to the Scientific Review Administrator responsible for the review. After the review has been completed, the principal investigator may contact the assigned Institute for the outcome of the review and information about the likelihood of funding. Finally, once the summary statement has been received, if the principal investigator feels that the review was flawed, he or she may contact the assigned institute for information about procedures to seek redress of his/her concerns. Further information about communicating concerns regarding the review of an application is available through the Office of Grants Inquiries, Division of Research Grants, National Institutes of Health, Bethesda, MD 20892, at (301) 496-7441, or through the various agency contacts listed on page 4.

B. GRANTEE RESPONSIBILITY AFTER AN AWARD

If a grant is awarded as the result of the application, the applicant organization becomes a grantee and assumes legal and financial accountability for the awarded funds and for the performance of the grant supported activities. The applicant organization is responsible for verifying the accuracy, validity, and conformity with the most current institutional guidelines of all the administrative, fiscal, and scientific information in the application, including the indirect cost rate. Deliberate withholding, falsification, or misrepresentation of information could result in administrative actions such as withdrawal of an application, the suspension and/or termination of an award, and debarment, as well as possible criminal penalties.

C. GOVERNMENT USE OF INFORMATION/PRIVACY ACT

In addition to using the information provided for reviewing applications and monitoring grantee performance, the PHS may use the information to identify candidates who may serve as ad hoc consultants, committee members, or National Advisory Council and Board members and to analyze costs of proposed grants.

The PHS maintains applications and grant records as part of a system of records defined by the Privacy Act: 09-25-0112, "Grants: Research, Research Training, Fellowship, and Construction Applications." The Privacy Act of 1974 (5 USC 552a) allows disclosures for "routine uses" and for permissible disclosures:

(1) To the cognizant audit agency for auditing;

(2) To a Congressional office in response to its inquiry regarding the record of an individual made at the request of that individual;

(3) To qualified experts, not within the definition of DHHS employees as prescribed in DHHS regulations (45 CFR 5b.2), for opinions as a part of the application review process;

(4) To a Federal agency, in response to its request, in connection with the letting of a contract or the issuance of a license, grant, or other benefit by the requesting agency, to the extent that the record is relevant and necessary to the requesting agency's decision on the matter;

(5) To organizations in the private sector with which the PHS has contracted for the purpose of collating, analyzing, aggregating, or otherwise refining records in a system. Relevant records will be disclosed to such a contractor, who will be required to maintain Privacy Act safeguards with respect to such records;

(6) To the applicant organization in connection with the review of an application or performance or administration under the terms and conditions of the award, or in connection with problems that might arise in performance or administration if an award is made;

(7) To the Department of Justice, to a court or other tribunal, or to another party before such tribunal, when one of the following is a party to litigation or has any interest in such litigation, and the DHHS determines that the use of such records by the Department of Justice, the tribunal, or the other party is relevant and necessary to the litigation and would help in the effective representation of the governmental party:

(a) The DHHS, or any component thereof;

(b) Any DHHS employee in his or her official capacity;

(c) Any DHHS employee in his or her individual capacity where the Department of Justice (or the DHHS, where it is authorized to do so) has agreed to represent the employee; or

(d) The United States or any agency thereof, where the DHHS determines that the litigation is likely to affect the DHHS or any of its components; and

(8) A record may also be disclosed for a research purpose, when the DHHS:

(a) Has determined that the use or disclosure does not violate legal or policy limitations under which the record was provided, collected, or obtained;

(b) Has determined that the research purpose (i) cannot be reasonably accomplished unless the record is provided in individually identifiable form, and (ii) warrants the risk to the privacy of the individual that additional exposure of the record might bring;

(c) Has secured a written statement attesting to the recipient's understanding of, and willingness to abide by, these provisions; and

(d) Has required the recipient to:

(i) Establish reasonable administrative, technical, and physical safeguards to prevent unauthorized use or disclosure of the record;

(ii) Remove or destroy the information that identifies the individual at the earliest time at which removal or destruction can be accomplished consistent with the purpose of the research project, unless the recipient has presented adequate justification of a research or health nature for retaining such information; and

(iii) Make no further use or disclosure of the record, except (a) in emergency circumstances affecting the health or safety of any individual, (b) for use in another research project, under these same conditions, and with written authorization of the DHHS, (c) for disclosure to a properly identified person for the purpose of an audit related to the research project, if information that would enable research subjects to be identified is removed or destroyed at the earliest opportunity consistent with the purpose of the audit, or (d) when required by law.

The Privacy Act also authorizes discretionary disclosures where determined appropriate by the PHS, including to law enforcement agencies; to the Congress acting within its legislative authority; to the Bureau of the Census; to the National Archives; to the General Accounting Office; pursuant to a court order; or as required to be disclosed by the Freedom of Information Act of 1974 (5 USC 552) and the associated DHHS regulations (45 CFR 5).

The PHS also maintains management information related to grants as part of another Privacy Act system of records: 09-25-0036, "Grants: IMPAC (Grant/Contract Information)."

D. INFORMATION AVAILABLE TO THE PRINCIPAL INVESTIGATOR/PROGRAM DIRECTOR

Under the provisions of the Privacy Act, principal investigators/program directors may request copies of records pertaining to their grant applications from the PHS component responsible for funding decisions. Principal investigators/program directors are given the opportunity under established procedures to request that the records be amended if they believe they are inaccurate, untimely, incomplete or irrelevant. If the PHS concurs, the records will be amended.

E. INFORMATION AVAILABLE TO THE GENERAL PUBLIC

The PHS makes information about awarded grants available to the public, including the title of the project, the grantee institution, the principal investigator/program director, and the amount of the award. The Description on form page 2 of a funded research grant application is sent to the National Technical Information Service (NTIS), U.S. Department of Commerce, where the information is used for the dissemination of scientific information and for scientific classification and program analysis purposes. These Descriptions are available to the public from the NTIS.

The Freedom of Information Act and implementing DHHS regulations (45 CFR Part 5) require the release of certain information about grants upon request, irrespective of the intended use of the information. Trade secrets and commercial, financial, or otherwise intrinsically valuable information that is obtained from a person or organization and that is privileged or confidential nformation may be withheld from disclosure. Information which, if disclosed, would be a clearly unwarranted invasion of personal privacy may also be withheld from disclosure. Although the grantee institution and the principal investigator/ program director will be consulted about any such release, the final determination will be made by the PHS. Generally available for release upon request, except as noted above, are: all funded grant applications *including* their derivative funded *noncompeting* supplemental grant applications; pending and funded *noncompeting continuation* applications; progress reports of grantees; and final reports of any review or evaluation of grantee performance conducted or caused to be conducted by the DHHS. Generally *not* available for release to the public are: **competing** grant applications (initial, competing continuation, and supplemental) for which awards have *not* been made; evaluative portions of site visit reports; and summary statements of findings and recommendations of review groups.

F. AUTHORIZATION

The PHS requests the information described in these instructions pursuant to its statutory authorities for awarding grants, contained in Sections 301(a) and 487 of the PHS Act, as amended (42 USC 241a and 42 USC 288). Therefore, such information must be submitted if an application is to receive due consideration for an award. Lack of sufficient information may hinder the PHS's ability to review an application and to monitor the grantee's performance.

G. RECOMBINANT DNA

The current NIH Guidelines for Research Involving Recombinant DNA Molecules and announcements of modifications and changes to the Guidelines are available from the Office of Recombinant DNA Activities, National Institutes of Health, Bethesda, MD 20892. All research involving recombinant DNA techniques that is supported by the DHHS must meet the requirements of these Guidelines. As defined by the Guidelines, recombinant DNA molecules are either: (1) molecules which are constructed outside living cells by joining natural or synthetic DNA segments to DNA molecules that can replicate in a living cell; or (2) DNA molecules that result from the replication of those described in (1) above.

Additional Instructions for PHS 398
Rev. 9/91

Form Approved Through 6/30/94
OMB No. 0925-0001

U.S. DEPARTMENT OF HEALTH
AND HUMAN SERVICES
Public Health Service

ADDITIONAL INSTRUCTIONS FOR PREPARING
RESEARCH CAREER DEVELOPMENT AWARD APPLICATIONS

The instructions and form pages in this kit are used with these additional instructions to request a K04 Research Career Development Award (RCDA). These instructions contain modifications to the instructions and forms, including a substitute Table of Contents page and the additional information requested of RCDA applicants. Follow both sets of instructions to avoid delays in the review of the application.

These instructions may not apply to all types of career development awards listed on page 6. To be sure the proper instructions and formats are used, contact the staff of the most relevant Institute. Applicants applying for any NIH K series award should obtain The K Awards book from the Office of Grants Inquiries, Division of Research Grants, National Institutes of Health, Bethesda, MD 20892.

Before preparing an application, review the RCDA guidelines, noting especially the eligibility requirements, award provisions, and review criteria. The guidelines, issued periodically in the *NIH Guide for Grants and Contracts*, are also available from the Office of Grants Inquiries. **While letters of reference are no longer required for the RCDA, they may be required for the other K series awards. Applicants are urged to consult with the appropriate PHS awarding component prior to submission.** Further information is available from the Office of Grants Inquiries.

The following instructions, items, and pages of the application are modified as indicated.

A. SPECIFIC INSTRUCTIONS– Forms

(Form Page 1)

Item 2a. Response to Specific Program Announcement. Indicate "Research Career Development Award."

Item 2b. Type of Grant Program. Insert K04.

Item 3. Principal Investigator/Program Director. Provide information on the candidate. Indicate in 3b the doctoral degree(s). If the candidate is not located at the applicant organization at the time the application is submitted the Mailing Address (Item 3e) and Telephone (Item 3h) should indicate where the applicant can be reached prior to the requested award date; items 3d, 3f, and 3g should reflect the candidate's projected position at the applicant organization.

Item 6. Dates of Entire Proposed Project Period. The project period must be 5 years. If the application involves a change of applicant organization for an active RCDA awardee, indicate the remaining time on the original 5-year award.

(Form Page 2)

Description. Provide an abstract of the whole application (candidate, environment, and research) not just the Research Plan. Include the candidate's immediate and long-term career

1

goals; how the award will make a difference in, and enhance, the candidate's development as an independent investigator; the institution's development plans and environment; and a brief abstract of the research project.

Personnel. Be certain to name the candidate's department head and senior staff member (if other than the department head) who will assume responsibility for the candidate's research career development at the applicant organization.

(Form Page 3)

TABLE OF CONTENTS

Replace the Research Grant Table of Contents page with the RCDA Substitute Page at the back of this addendum. Follow the instructions below for verifying citizenship.

Citizenship. Candidates for an award must be citizens or non-citizen nationals of the United States or its possessions and territories, or must have been lawfully admitted to the United States for permanent residence at the time of application. Permanent residents must submit with the application a notarized statement indicating that the candidate has an Alien Registration Receipt Card, and that the form number of the card is either 1-551 or 1-151.

(Form Page 4)

DETAILED BUDGET FOR INITIAL BUDGET PERIOD

Only the candidate's base salary up to $50,000 and an additional amount for related fringe benefits may be requested as direct costs. Salary levels are subject to change; current information on salaries is available from the Office of Grants Inquiries.

Personnel. Base the candidate's request on a full-time 12-month appointment, following the salary and fringe benefits guidelines in the RCDA program announcement and the instructions for personnel. Do **not** list other individuals involved on the project.

(Form Page 5)

BUDGET FOR ENTIRE PROPOSED PROJECT PERIOD

Provide separate estimates for salary and fringe benefits for each year.

Justification. Provide information to support the total salary and fringe benefits to be provided the awardee in the first year, and any increases in future years. The total salary includes the salary requested in this application and any supplementation by the applicant organization. List the following details:

(1) How the total salary amount for the first year was derived, showing the relevant parts of the salary structure including ranges of salaries being paid to comparable staff members;

(2) If supplementation is proposed, the supplemental amount and the source(s) of that supplemental support;

(3) The total **current** professional income of the candidate, and the source(s) of that income;

(4) The applicant organization's **current** contribution for fringe benefits;

(5) Whether or not professional fees will be generated by the candidate from clinical practice, professional consultation, or other comparable activities, describing the full circumstances, amounts, and plans of the applicant organization relating to the disposition of such fees; and

(6) The basis for any increases requested in future years, including percentages if a recurring annual increase is anticipated.

Provide at the end of the justification the typed name, title, and signature and date signed by the official who is responsible for the application of the salary scale to professional personnel within the organization. Usually such an individual is the graduate school dean, the medical school

2

dean, or the official with comparable responsibility within other types of organizations. "Per" signatures are not acceptable.

BIOGRAPHICAL SKETCH

Complete this page only for the candidate.

Education. Give the month as well as the year on which any degrees were conferred. For nondegree education, indicate the time period covered.

Research and/or Professional Experience. Substitute these instructions for those on the form page. Identify each heading. If necessary, use more than two pages.

1. **Employment.** Start with the first position held following the baccalaureate and give a consecutive record to date. Indicate the department and organization, department head or supervisor, rank, tenured or non-tenured, status (full- or part-time), and inclusive dates. Where applicable, include information on military service, internships, residencies, research assistantships, fellowships, etc.

2. **Honors.** List academic and professional honors.

3. **Professional Societies.** Identify professional societies and related organizations in which membership has been held within the last 10 years, giving dates.

4. **Publications.** In chronological order, list the candidate's **entire bibliography** with titles and complete references. Identify the publications that accompany the application (up to six may be included in the Appendix). See Item 3, Progress Report/Preliminary Studies, below.

Other Support. Complete this page only for the candidate.

Resources and Environment. Complete this section carefully. The information provided is critical to the review process.

B. SPECIFIC INSTRUCTIONS– Research Plan

Research Plan.

3. **Progress Report/Preliminary Studies.** A progress report is required only when the application involves a change of awardee organization for an active RCDA investigator. In preparing the report, disregard that part of the instructions asking for a list of professional personnel involved with the project.

8. **Consortium/Contractual Arrangements.** If, during the 5-year period, the candidate proposes to spend a period of time at another organization, provide a detailed explanation. If this period is longer than 3 months, submit a copy of a letter or other evidence to ensure that satisfactory arrangements have been made with the other organization. A description of the fiscal and administrative arrangements is not needed.

10. **References (where required).** A list of individuals submitting letters of reference must be included here. Provide the name, title, and institutional affiliation for each individual.

Specialized RCDA Information

This information is required for all RCDA applicants and should follow the Research Plan. The candidate prepares Item 1; the sponsoring department prepares Items 2 and 3.

1. **Candidate's Plans**

   a. **Career Plans.** Provide a brief summary of your immediate and long-term career objectives and plans. Explain how an RCDA would make a difference in, and enhance, your development as an independent investigator.

   b. **Other Activities.** Describe each of the activities, except research, to be engaged in during the proposed award period (5 years). Include a percentage of time involvement for each activity by year and explain how the activity is related to your research career development.

2. **Applicant Organization's Plans**
Describe fully the applicant organization's plans for the candidate's support and research career development for the entire period of the proposed award. Include a description of the proposed status of the candidate in the department and his/her relationship to colleagues.

If applicable, describe the organization's plans for the candidate's supervision, guidance, counseling, or any other formal and informal training. Describe opportunities for interaction with investigators in other departments and, if appropriate, at other organizations.

Explain in detail how the award will make a difference in and enhance the candidate's research career development. Include a description of the candidate's teaching load for the **current** academic year, including number and types of courses or seminars; clinical duties, including number of patients currently seen and professional consultations; committee and administrative assignments; and proportion of time currently available for research. Provide at the end of the

organization's plan the signature of and date signed by the head of the department or departmental subdivision or appropriate comparable organizational unit. "Per" signatures are not acceptable.

3. **Institutional Commitment**

A letter should be submitted by the candidate's department chair describing plans for the candidate at the conclusion of the RCDA and indicating how he/she would spend **the next five years** if he/she received an award versus how the time would be spent if an award was not received. **These remarks should emphasize how the award will contribute to the candidate's research career.**

CHECKLIST.

Indirect Costs. Indirect costs on RCDAs will be awarded at 8 percent of total direct costs.

C. SPECIFIC INSTRUCTIONS– Appendix

No more than six publications and manuscripts accepted for publication should be submitted with **New** applications. Do not submit abstracts or unpublished theses.

Instructions for PHS 398
Rev. 9/91

Form Approved Through 6/30/94
OMB No. 0925-0001

U.S. DEPARTMENT OF HEALTH AND HUMAN SERVICES
Public Health Service

ADDITIONAL INSTRUCTIONS FOR PREPARING INSTITUTIONAL NATIONAL RESEARCH SERVICE AWARD APPLICATIONS

The instructions and form pages in this kit are used with these additional instructions to request competing (new, competing continuation, and supplemental) support under the PHS Institutional National Research Service Award (NRSA) Program. These instructions contain modifications to the instructions and forms, including three substitute form pages (the table of contents page and both budget pages) and instructions for the Research Training Program plan. Follow both sets of instructions to avoid delays in the review of applications.

Applicants are urged to consult with the appropriate PHS awarding component prior to submission. In addition, before preparing an application, review the NRSA program announcement, noting especially the eligibility requirements, award provisions, payback service provisions, and review criteria. Program announcements, which are issued periodically in the *NIH Guide for Grants and Contracts*, are also available from the appropriate PHS awarding component. **When individuals start training under an Institutional NRSA, they must provide written assurance to the Secretary, DHHS, that they will meet the payback service requirements.** Applicant organization officials responsible for recruitment of trainees should familiarize themselves with the terms of the service requirements and explain them to prospective training candidates before or at the time an appointment at the institution is offered. Further details on policies governing the NRSA program can be found in the National Research Service Award Guidelines for Individual Awards - Institutional Grants, as amended. This docu-

ment is usually available at grantee offices of sponsored programs or equivalent offices. The applicant organization should be certain to have the latest edition of these guidelines.

The following instructions, items, and pages of the application are modified as indicated below.

A. SPECIFIC INSTRUCTIONS– Forms

(Form Page 1)

Item 2a. Response to Specific Request for Applications (RFA) or Program Announcement (PA). Indicate "Institutional National Research Service Award" and include the specific PHS awarding component and specialized program area, if applicable.

Item 2b. Type of Grant Program. Refer to Page 10.

Item 4. Human Subjects. If the applicant organization has an approved Assurance of Compliance on file with OPRR but, at the time of application, plans for the involvement of human subjects are so indefinite that Institutional Review Board (IRB) review and approval are not feasible, check the box marked "YES" and insert "indefinite" at Item 4a. If an award is made, human subjects may **not** be involved until a certification of the date of IRB approval or a designation of exemption has been submitted to the PHS awarding component.

1

In many instances, trainees supported by institutional training grants will be participating in research supported by research project grants for which the IRB review of human subjects is already complete or an exemption is already designated. This review or exemption designation is sufficient, providing the research would not be substantially modified by the participation of a trainee. The appropriate grants must be identified along with their IRB review dates or exemption designation. If space is insufficient in Item 4, indicate at 4a "Sec. C5" and provide the information under 5 in the Research Plan.

Item 5. Vertebrate Animals. If the applicant organization has an approved Animal Welfare Assurance on file with OPRR but, at the time of application, plans for the involvement of vertebrate animals are so indefinite that Institutional Animal Care and Use Committee (IACUC) review and approval are not feasible, check the box marked "YES" and insert "indefinite" at Item 5a. If an award is made, vertebrate animals may **not** be involved until a verification of the date of IACUC approval has been submitted to the PHS awarding component.

In many instances, trainees supported by institutional training grants will be participating in research supported by research project grants for which the IACUC review is already complete. This review is sufficient, providing the research would not be substantially modified by the participation of a trainee. The appropriate grants must be identified along with their IACUC review dates. If space is insufficient in Item 5, indicate at 5a "Sec. C6" and provide the information under 6 in the Research Plan.

Item 6. Dates of Entire Proposed Project Period. The usual starting date for an institutional NRSA is July 1, but there are other possible starting dates. Consult the review and award schedules on page 8 in the general instructions. A few PHS awarding components restrict receipt and review dates to once a year. **Applicants are strongly encouraged to contact appropriate awarding component staff before submitting an application.**

Item 10. Inventions and Patents. Not applicable.

(Form Page 2)

Description. Summarize the essence and major features of the program. Include research areas and disciplines, levels of training, numbers and background experience of trainees, and primary facilities.

(Form Page 3)

TABLE OF CONTENTS

Use the substitute Table of Contents page in this addendum.

(Form Page 4)

DETAILED BUDGET FOR INITIAL BUDGET PERIOD

Use the substitute page in this addendum and follow the instructions below. Refer to the NRSA program announcement or consult the PHS awarding component for current allowable costs and stipend levels. Provide information where possible on the substitute form page 4 with additional details starting in the budget Justification block on substitute form page 5.

Stipends. Enter the number of trainees and total stipend amount for each trainee category as appropriate. If a category contains different stipend levels, e.g., for varying levels of postdoctoral experience and/or varying appointment periods, itemize. Enter the total stipends for all categories.

Tuition, Fees, and Insurance. Explain in detail the composition of this item. Itemize tuition, individual fees, and medical insurance. If tuition varies, e.g., in state, out-of-state, student status, identify these separately. Tuition at the postdoctoral level is limited to that required for specified courses. Tuition and fees (including self only health insurance) may be requested only to the extent that the same resident or nonresident tuition and fees are charged to regular non-Federally supported students.

Trainee Travel. State the purpose of any travel, giving the number of trips involved, the destinations, and the number of individuals for

2

whom funds are requested, bearing in mind that PHS policy requires less than first-class air travel be used. Justify foreign travel in detail, describing its importance to the training experience.

Training Related Expenses. Funds to defray other costs of training, such as staff salaries, consultant costs, equipment, research supplies, staff travel, etc., are requested as a lump sum based on the predetermined amount, specified in the program announcement, per predoctoral and postdoctoral trainee. Give the number of trainees at each predetermined rate, and enter the total dollar figure. No further itemization or explanation is required.

(Form Page 5)

BUDGET FOR ENTIRE PROPOSED PROJECT PERIOD

Use the substitute page in this addendum.

(Form Additional Pages)

BIOGRAPHICAL SKETCH

Include sketches, not to exceed two pages each, for all professional personnel contributing to the training program. Assemble sketches with the program director first and others following in alphabetical order.

OTHER SUPPORT

Follow these instructions instead of those on the form page. Provide a table that lists, for each participating faculty member, active and pending **research** support. Include all Federal, non-Federal, and institutional research grant and contract support. If none, state "none." Include the source of support, the grant number and title, dates of entire project period, and annual direct costs. If part of a larger project, identify the principal investigator and provide the above data for both the parent grant and the subproject. **Training** grant support is to be listed in the Research Training Program Plan, (See **Background** below).

RESOURCES AND ENVIRONMENT

Describe the facilities and resources which will be used in the proposed training program. Indicate in what ways the applicant organization will support the program (e.g., supplementation of stipends).

B. SPECIFIC INSTRUCTIONS– Research Training Program Plan

Research Training Program Plan

After the Introduction for **Revised** or **Supplemental** applications, follow the outline suggested below in describing the Research Training Program Plan. **Do not exceed 25 pages of narrative overall for sections 1-4.** Much of the information requested may be provided in tabular form, which will not be counted toward the page limitation.

Before completing the training plan, you are strongly encouraged to contact the appropriate PHS awarding component, which may have some further advice or suggestions for organizing the relevant data into particular formats.

1. Background

Give the rationale for the proposed research training program, relevant background history, and the need for the research training proposed. Indicate how the proposed program relates to current training activities.

Summarize the research training activities of the major participating unit(s) and department(s) represented in the proposed program. Give the current number of faculty members in each unit/department, as well as the total numbers of current predoctoral and postdoctoral students.

In a table, list all current and pending training support available to the participating faculty and department(s). Include funding source, complete identifying number, title of the training program, name of the program director, project period, number of trainee positions (predoctoral and postdoctoral), and amount of the award. For each grant listed, name those participating faculty members who are also named in **this** application.

2. Program Plan

a. Program Direction.

Describe the program director's relevant scientific background, research, experience in research training, and qualifications for providing leadership for the program. Indicate the program director's percent of effort in the proposed program.

Describe the administrative structure of the program and the distribution of responsibilities within it, including the means by which the program director will obtain continuing advice with respect to the operation of the program.

b. Program Faculty.

List each training faculty member, his/her primary departmental affiliation, role, and percent of effort in the proposed program.

Describe each faculty member's research that is relevant to this program and indicate how trainees will participate in this research.

Describe the extent to which participating faculty members cooperated, interacted, and collaborated in the past, including joint publications and joint sponsorship of student research.

In a table, for each faculty member participating in this application, list all past and current students for whom the faculty member has served or is serving as thesis advisor or sponsor (limited to the past 10 years). For each student listed, indicate (1) whether training was at the predoctoral or postdoctoral level; (2) the training period; (3) the institution and degree received prior to entry into training, including date; (4) title of the research project; and (5) for **past** students, their current positions, and for **current** students, their source of support. In **Competing Continuation** applications, asterisk those trainees who were or are supported by this training grant. Individuals who were trained by proposed participating faculty members at sites other than the applicant organization may be included but should be specifically identified. For **New** applications, list representative recent publications of some of the above students. For **Competing Continuation** applications, publications of past trainees supported by this grant, provided in the Progress Report, will suffice.

c. Proposed Training.

Describe the proposed training program. Give the level and number of trainees. For postdoctoral trainees, the proposed distribution by degree (M.D., Ph.D., etc.) should be provided. Describe course work and research opportunities, the extent to which trainees will participate directly in research, the duration of training (i.e., usual period of time required to complete the training offered), and the fields in which trainees will be qualified upon completion of training.

Indicate how the individual disciplinary and/or departmental components in the program are integrated and coordinated for the program and for an individual trainee's experience.

For training programs emphasizing research training for clinicians, describe the interactions with basic science departments and scientists. In addition, include plans for ensuring that the training of these physicians will provide a substantive foundation for a competitive research career. Generally, a minimum of two years of research training is required for all postdoctoral trainees with health professional degrees. Describe fully any trainee access to and responsibility for patients, including percent of effort.

Provide representative examples of individual trainee programs. Include curricula, degree requirements, didactic courses, laboratory experiences, qualifying examinations, and other training

4

activities, such as seminars, journal clubs, etc. Describe how the preceptor and research problems are chosen, how each trainee's program will be guided, and how the trainee's performance will be monitored and evaluated.

d. Responsible Conduct of Research. Describe plans to provide trainees with instruction on scientific integrity and ethical principles in research. Include a description of both formal (courses, seminars, etc.) and informal training activities that will be incorporated into the proposed training program.

e. Trainee Candidates. Describe recruitment plans, including the sources and availability of trainees. Give the qualifications of prospective trainees and the criteria and procedures by which trainees will be selected. Clearly indicate which applicants would be eligible for training grant support based on citizenship or permanent residency status.

In a table, for each participating department/unit, for each of the past five years, give the number of individuals who have formally applied for training, the number of individuals who have been offered admission, the number who have entered training, the number who have completed the intended training or are currently in training, and the number who have left the program. Indicate whether these individuals were applying for predoctoral or postdoctoral training, and for postdoctoral fellows, give their degrees (M.D., Ph.D., etc.).

3. Recruitment of Individuals from Underrepresented Racial/Ethnic Groups

The policy of the NIH and ADAMHA is to promote broad and systematic efforts to recruit individuals from minority groups currently underrepresented in biomedical and behavioral research. National Research Service Award programs are intended to attract and train individuals to pursue independent careers as investigators. Accomplishments of NRSA programs in these areas with respect to minority groups will ensure that minority scientists are progressively better represented in the National research effort.

Describe the program's plans and experiences regarding the recruitment and training of Blacks, Hispanics, Native Americans, Pacific Islanders, or members of other ethnic or racial groups which have been found to be underrepresented in biomedical or behavioral research Nationally.

Applications without such specific plans may be deferred.

Describe steps to be taken to identify and recruit students from minority groups that are now underrepresented Nationally in the biomedical and behavioral sciences. Specific efforts to be undertaken by this training program should be delineated. It may be appropriate to include efforts of the medical school, graduate school, and/or university at large, if these impact directly on those made by the program. Those efforts by the institution do **not** preclude a plan specific to the proposed program.

Provide recruitment statistics indicating the number of minority individuals who applied to the program and/or participating units in each of the past three years. Give the number of minority candidates offered admission and the number who entered the program. For those who entered the program, indicate their current status (e.g., in training, graduated or completed training, left the program). Give the source of support for these students. For **competing continuation** applications, indicate students who received support from this training grant.

For trainees from underrepresented minority groups who have completed the training program, provide statistics on subsequent career development, including postgraduate training and current positions.

4. Progress Report (Competing Continuation Applications Only)

Briefly describe the accomplishments of the training program. State the period covered.

Provide a table documenting, for each year of the current project period, the program's actual commitment of awarded trainee positions. Give (1) the total number of positions awarded in each year; (2) the number of predoctoral trainees appointed and months of support committed; and (3) the number of postdoctoral trainees appointed, with what degrees, at what levels, and for how many months. Indicate and explain any trainee positions that were not filled.

Provide a table listing all trainees who were or are supported by this training grant. (Where applicable, provide data for the past 10 years.) For each student, give (1) the name; (2) the year of entry into the training program, prior institution, and degree at entry; (3) the source of support during each year of training (e.g., this training grant, another [specify] training grant, research grant, university fellowship, individual [specify] fellowship, etc.); (4) the research mentor; (5) the research topic; and (6) for trainees who have completed the program, their current positions and institutional affiliations. Where possible for past trainees, describe the extent of their current involvement in research, including research grant support and representative recent publications. The information in this table will be used to track the pattern of support of trainees and the subsequent research career development of former trainees.

Also, explain why any postdoctoral trainee with a health professional degree, who was appointed to the grant during the most recent award period, has received less than two years of research training. This explanation should appear in the narrative section of the Progress Report.

Give a brief summary of the research conducted by each trainee supported during the period covered and list all publications that resulted from the work done during training.

Describe any specific effects of this training program on curriculum and/or research directions.

Describe how the funds provided under Training Related Expenses were utilized to benefit the program.

5. Human Subjects

As indicated earlier in these instructions for Item 4 on the Face Page, where appropriate include a list of already reviewed research project grants and their IRB review dates or exemption designations.

6. Vertebrate Animals

As indicated earlier in these instructions for Item 5 on the Face Page, where appropriate include a list of already reviewed research project grants and their IACUC review dates.

CHECKLIST

Indirect Costs. Indirect costs under Institutional NRSAs other than those issued to State or local government agencies will be awarded at 8 percent of total direct costs (exclusive of tuition and related fees). Equipment is also excluded on those training grants where Training Related Expenses are not calculated on a lump-sum basis, such as the MARC Honors Undergraduate Research Training Program. State and local government agencies will receive awards at their full indirect cost rates.

C. SPECIFIC INSTRUCTIONS– Appendix

Appendix material is generally not needed with training grant applications. Oversized documents, brochures, and catalogues may be exceptions. Five collated sets should be submitted.

6

Appendix 2

Extramural Support Mechanisms

RESEARCH GRANT PROGRAMS

The NIH activity code is included in parentheses after the title of each type of grant.

Research Project Grant—Traditional (R01)

Description

This award is made to an eligible institution on behalf of a principal investigator (PI) for a circumscribed biomedical or behavioral project related to the investigator's interests and competence.

Comments

Awards are made to nonprofit and for-profit organizations and institutions, both domestic and foreign; to government agencies; and rarely to individuals. Any qualified scientist may apply. Access to necessary facilities is essential, as well as assurances that grant funds will be properly managed. Projects must be health related. There is no limitation on the number or dollar value of awards that can be made to an institution generally, or to an institution on behalf of one individual.

Awarding Units

All NIH institutes offer R01 support with the exception of FIC.

Program Project Grant (P01)

Description

This is an award to an institution on behalf of a senior PI for the support of a broadly based, usually multidisciplinary, long-term research program with a clearly defined, unifying central theme. It involves the efforts of a group of investigators, each responsible for a research project(s) and/or shared resources (core units) contributing to the overall program objective. Usually a minimum of three meritorious research projects is necessary to launch a viable program.

Comments

Guidelines and policies governing the preparation, review, and funding of these applications are not uniform among the NIH institutes and may differ due to philosophy, fiscal constraints, and programmatic management. Therefore, it is essential to contact program staff during the early planning stage. Some institutes have brochures outlining requirements for these awards, as well as instructions for preparing applications. Most institutes have placed a dollar ceiling on a P01 award, usually in the range of $500,000 to $1 million per year, direct costs only. Applications exceeding the specific institute limit will be returned without review. Several institutes use an RFA to solicit applications in specific program areas. With few exceptions, peer review of applications is managed by institute staff utilizing any one or a combination of site visit teams, ad hoc committees, or standing program project committees. Although the P01 is considered an unsolicited, investigator-initiated mechanism, investigators can avoid grief and delays by consulting ICD staff before preparing an application. Awards are not made to foreign institutions.

Awarding Units

All NIH awarding units offer this type of support with the exception of NEI, NLM, NCRR, and FIC.

U.S.–Japan Cooperative Medical Science Program (R22)

Description

The program is intended to support research, in a limited number of medical problem areas, for the benefit of the people of Asia.

Comments

The program is confined to six research areas: cholera, leprosy, malnutrition, parasitic diseases (schistosomiasis and filariasis), tuberculosis, and certain viral diseases (primarily rabies and dengue hemorrhagic fever). Application, peer review, and award procedures are identical to the R01 program.

Awarding Units

NIAID, NICHD, and NIDDK.

First Independent Research Support and Transition (FIRST Award (R29)

Description

This award is designed to provide a sufficient initial period of research support for newly independent biomedical investigators, working in the basic or clinical sciences, to develop their research skills and ideas. It is a nonrenewable, five-year award with total direct costs not to exceed $350,000 for all years or $100,000 in any one year.

Comment

An eligible individual must not be in training status at the time of award nor have been PI on a previously peer-reviewed, PHS research project. Exceptions are an R03 (Small Grant Program) or an R15 (Academic Research Enhancement Award) or certain career (K) awards directed principally to physicians, dentists, and veterinarians with little research experience. Recipients of a FIRST award must commit at least 50 percent time and effort to the project in each twelve-month budget period. Carryover of unobligated funds from one budget period to the next is allowed, as is an extension of the project period for one year without additional funds. Only one application can be submitted per receipt date. Concurrent submission of other types of grant applications is not permitted. However, after an award is made, the latter restriction no longer applies so long as the 50 percent commitment to the FIRST award is maintained. A FIRST award may not be used to supplement a project already supported by PHS funds. Applications are peer reviewed by DRG study sections. Awards are not made to foreign institutions.

Awarding Units

All NIH awarding units are authorized to use this mechanism. All do except FIC.

Outstanding Investigator Grant (OIG) (R35)

Description

This award recognizes investigators for their established preeminence and productivity. The purpose is to provide stable, renewable, financial support and research flexibility for periods up to seven years, and to encourage long-term projects of unusual research potential.

Comment

A minimum of ten years of previous, consecutive, peer-reviewed support is required. There are no age restrictions. A letter of intent including a curriculum vitae, listing of research support received from all sources, and a three-page description of research accomplishments is to be submitted. Letters are reviewed and those approved are invited to complete an abbreviated PHS 398 application not to exceed five pages of text. There must be evidence of institutional support and a minimum of 75 percent time commitment. Applications are evaluated by an institute-managed, ad hoc peer review committee. Contact staff for more information.

Awarding Units

NCI and NIA.

Method to Extend Research In Time (MERIT) Award (R37)

Description

The objective of this award is to provide long-term, stable support of up to ten years to outstanding investigators. No special application is required.

Comments

Awards are based on the results of normal study section review of competing R01 applications. Selections are made by staff and advisory councils on the basis of an excellent priority score, recommended support for five years, and the scientific achievements in a research area of special interest. After the initial five years, awardees must submit an eight-page progress report, a one-page abstract of future plans, and a budget. Staff and advisory councils review this material and approve extensions for periods up to an additional five years. Carryover of unexpended funds is allowed throughout the entire period of the award.

Awarding Units

All awarding units participating in the R01 program are authorized to use this mechanism. The NINDS uses a similar selection process but the award is designated the Senator Jacob Javits Neuroscience Award.

Small Business Innovation Research Grants (SBIR) Phase I (R43)

Description

The SBIR mechanism supports projects at small businesses having the expertise to contribute to the mission of the NIH. The purpose of Phase I projects is to establish the technical merit and feasibility of research and development ideas that may ultimately lead to a commercial product(s) or service(s). Awards normally do not exceed six months or $50,000 in total costs.

Comments

The objectives are to stimulate technical innovation in the private sector and to encourage participation by women, minority, and disadvantaged persons in such endeavors. Small businesses are defined as those independently owned, operated for profit, not dominant in a field, and with no more than 500 employees.

Awarding Units

All NIH awarding units with the exception of the FIC.

Small Business Innovation Research Grants (SBIR) Phase II (R44)

Description

A Phase II award supports in-depth development of research and development ideas whose feasibility have been established in Phase I and which are likely to result in commercial products or services. Awards normally do not exceed two years or $500,000 in total costs.

Comments

Same as above. NIH publishes a booklet on the SBIR program providing all relevant details such as requirements and application preparation. A copy of this omnibus solicitation can be obtained by writing to:

> **SBIR Solicitation Office**
> **13687 Baltimore Ave.**
> **Laurel, MD 20707-5083**
> **(301) 206–9385**

Awarding Units

All NIH awarding units with the exception of FIC.

CENTER PROGRAMS

Applications generally are solicited via RFAs. These are usually five-year awards with maximum annual dollar amounts, in most, but not all cases, prescribed by the sponsoring ICD. Peer review is managed by ICD review staff using any one or a combination of ad hoc committees, site visit teams, or standing review committees. All NIH awarding units support at least one type of center except FIC.

Exploratory Grants (P20)

Description

The purpose is to support planning and exploratory studies that usually lead to specialized or comprehensive centers.

Comments

Funds are intended for planning new programs, expansion or modification of existing resources, and feasibility studies for the development of interdisciplinary programs of special significance to NIH. For more information, contact awarding units.

Awarding Units

In FY 1991, NIA, NIDCD, NCHGR, NCNR, and NINDS.

Center Core Grants (P30)

Description

This type of award is intended to provide shared, core facilities to enhance the productivity of an active group of investigators with their own research support, obtained through other mechanisms, e.g., R01s, and who work in areas related to the interest(s) of the sponsoring institute.

Comments

Examples of core units would be an administrative core to ensure sufficient support services for the group; biostatistics core to help with research design and data management and analysis; various laboratory cores to provide scientific expertise and analytic capability, e.g., molecular biology, immunology, etc.; instrumentation cores to maintain, develop, and conduct analyses with research equipment; clinical cores to recruit, process, and conduct tests on patients used in research studies (one institute gives as an example the use of mobile units for clinical studies involving the elderly and handicapped); and many others that a creative group might propose to satisfy a need. Core grants often supply funds to hire new faculty and for pilot research projects. They usually do not fund research projects eligible for support via other NIH grant mechanisms. There is a remarkable diversity of requirements identified by the various NIH awarding units for these awards. These are outlined in RFAs and brochures which can be obtained from the institutes.

Awarding Units

NIA, NIAID, NIAMS, NCI, NICHD, NIDDK, NIEHS, NEI, and NCHGR.

Animal Resources (P40)

Description

This is an award to support animal resources available to all qualified investigators within an institution or geographic area without regard to the disciplinary or disease orientation of their research activities.

Comment

These grants provide a central resource for many investigators studying problems related to the program interests of many NIH funding components. The NCRR should be contacted for details.

Awarding Units
NCRR.

Biotechnology Resources (P41)

Description

This mechanism supports biotechnology resources available to all qualified investigators within an institution or geographic area without regard to the disciplinary or disease orientation of their research activities.

Comments

These grants provide a central resource for many investigators studying problems related to the program interests of many NIH funding components. Examples are computer centers, mass spectrometry centers, electron microscopy centers, etc. The NCRR should be contacted for details.

Awarding Units
NCRR.

Hazardous Substances Basic Research Grants Program (P42)

Description

The award supports basic research directed toward understanding and attenuating public health effects resulting from exposure to hazardous substances.

Comments

This is a special program authorized under Superfund legislation. Applications should describe a broadly based, multidisciplinary research effort which may include engineering, hydrogeology, ecology, and epidemiology linked to basic bi-omedical sciences. Each research project is generally under the leadership of an established investigator. Core resources to support the group are permitted, including an administrative structure for effective coordination. For more information, contact NIEHS.

Awarding Units

NIEHS.

Specialized Centers (P50)

Description

This is an award to an institution on behalf of a senior PI, usually for the support of a multidisciplinary, clinical and basic, long-term research program with a central theme directed at a special program interest(s) of an institute. It involves the efforts of a group of investigators, each responsible for a research project(s) or shared resources (core units) contributing to the overall program objective. The intent is to concentrate research effort and resources on areas of high program relevance to an institute, e.g., specific disease states.

Comments

These are similar to program projects except for the requirement, in most but not all cases, of a clinical orientation. Also applications are solicited by RFAs that specify conditions of an award and other necessary information. Such centers usually represent an interactive network of specialized expertise committed to information exchange and rapid dissemination of research results.

Awarding Units

NIA, NIAID, NIAMS, NCI, NICHD, NIDCD, NIDR, NIDDK, NEI, NIGMS, NHLBI, NINDS, NCHGR, NCNR, and NLM.

Primate Research Centers (P51)

Description

This award supports multidisciplinary and multicategorical core research programs using primate animals. It involves maintaining a large and varied primate colony that is available to affiliated, collaborative, and visiting investigators for basic and applied biomedical research and training.

Comments

The NCRR should be contacted for details.

Awarding Units

NCRR.

Comprehensive Centers (P60)

Description

The P60 is an award to support a multidisciplinary, coordinated, disease-oriented program involving laboratory and clinical research. Depending on the sponsoring ICD's requirements, other activities could be included, such as research training; demonstration projects; continuing education programs for medical and allied health professionals; community education, screening, and counseling programs; and dissemination of information to the general public about the diagnosis and treatment of specific diseases or disorders.

Comments

These awards are structured in different ways. Some institutes require a broad spectrum of activities to be supported by this type of grant. In other cases, the award is considered an enhancement of ongoing support by the addition of, for example, demonstration and education research components to a Specialized Center.

Awarding Units

NIA, NIAMS, NIDCD, NIDDK, and NHLBI.

General Clinical Research Centers (M01)

Description

The M01 is an award made to an institution for the support of a discrete unit of hospital beds to be used by investigators to conduct studies on a wide range of human diseases using the full spectrum of the biomedical sciences.

Comments

These are specialized facilities with their own professional director, paramedical staff, biostatistician, laboratories, diet kitchen, research nursing, and dietary personnel. The NCRR should be contacted for details.

Awarding Units

NCRR.

CAREER DEVELOPMENT PROGRAMS

"Several types of career awards are available to research and academic institutions on behalf of scientists with clear research potential, but who require additional training and experience in a productive scientific environment in preparation for careers in independent research in the health sciences . . . While some of the programs are either trans-NIH in scope or are offered by most of the awarding components, a few are unique to a particular NIH component." These are quotes from an NIH publication, *K Awards*, which describes such programs in considerable detail. The booklet can be obtained from:

Office of Grant Inquiries
Room 449, Westwood Bldg.
DRG, NIH
Bethesda, MD 20892
(301) 496–7441

Interested applicants should contact NIH staff before submitting applications.

Special Emphasis Research Career Award (SERCA) (K01)

Description

This nonrenewable, five-year award is intended to encourage researchers, at an early stage of their careers, to acquire in-depth, multidisciplinary basic and clinical research experience in scientific areas designated by the sponsoring institute.

Comments

Candidates are nominated by domestic institutions who must also provide the release time, resources, and a sponsor to oversee the proposed development program. Candidates must hold a Ph.D. or M.D. or equivalent professional degree (D.V.M., D.D.S., D.O., etc.) and have a minimum of two years of research experience. A minimum of 75 percent of an awardee's time must be devoted to research. A maximum base salary of up to $50,000 is allowed with supplementation from nonfederal funds permitted. Annual research costs of between $8,000 and $20,000 are included in the award. Applications are peer reviewed by institute-managed committees.

Awarding Units and Emphasis Areas

NIA	Nutritional and metabolic factors in aging
	Rehabilitation and aging: Biomedical and psychological perspectives
	Social and behavioral scientists in behavioral geriatrics research
	Research in geriatric otolaryngology
NCRR	Laboratory animal science (D.V.M. required)

Research Career Development Award (RCDA) (K04)

Description

The RCDA is a nonrenewable, five-year salary grant to enhance the research capability of young scientists with outstanding research potential for careers of independent research in the biomedical sciences.

Comments

The purpose is to provide investigators who have attained some research accomplishments additional time in a productive environment to establish an independent research program. Candidates must be nominated by domestic institutions and are expected to devote at least 80 percent of their time to research. They should normally have five years of postdoctoral research experience, including two years as PI of a peer-reviewed grant from NIH or other sources. Awarding units will not make an award unless candidates have support for the research proposed in the application. The institution must make a commitment to provide the required research time, assurance that research support is available, and describe plans for the candidate's postaward future. Candidates with tenure, substantial publication records, or research support requiring a major time commitment are usually considered ineligible. Applications are referred for peer review to the DRG study section which reviewed other grant applications from the candidate. The maximum base salary is up to $50,000 for twelve months' full-time effort with supplementation from nonfederal funds permitted.

Awarding Units

All awarding units except NEI, NCNR, NCRR, NLM, and FIC.

Academic/Teacher Award (K07)

Description

This nonrenewable award is designed for investigators who wish to introduce or improve a curriculum to enhance the institutional research environment or the individual's own career in a medical or scientific specialty designated by an NIH institute.

Comments

Awardees must hold an academic appointment at the applicant institution and commit at least 50 percent time to developing, improving, and implementing a curriculum to enrich the research environment. Applications are peer reviewed by institute-managed committees.

Awarding Units and Emphasis Areas

NIA　　　The Geriatric Leadership Academic Award: Three-year awards to develop research and training programs in aging.

The Geriatric Academic Award: Five-year awards to recruit and support individuals with high potential for academic and/or research careers in geriatric medicine and related clinical areas.

NIAID　　The Allergic Diseases Academic Award: Five-year awards to permit institutions to obtain academic leadership and develop academic positions relating to allergic diseases.

NIEHS　　The Mid-Career Development Award—Environmental Toxicology: These are three-year awards to encourage individuals to enter careers in environmental toxicology.

The Environmental/Occupational Medicine Academic Award: Awards are for the dual purpose of improving the quality of environmental/occupational medicine curricula and of fostering research careers in medicine.

NCI　　　The Preventive Oncology Program (Academic Award): Awards are for development or improvement of research and curricula concerned with the etiology and primary prevention of cancer.

NHLBI　　Academic Award in Systemic and Pulmonary Vascular Disease: Awards are for the purpose of stimulating development of clinical, educational, and research programs and to promote professional development of the awardee in vascular medicine.

NCNR　　Academic Investigator Award—Nursing: Awards to enhance the research environment in schools of nursing and to strengthen the research careers of nurse scientists.

Clinical Investigator Award (CIA) K08)

Description

This is a nonrenewable award designed to provide the opportunity for promising clinically trained individuals to develop into independent biomedical investigators. It enables candidates to investigate a well-defined problem under a sponsor (or sponsors) competent to provide guidance in the chosen area of research. The award is intended to facilitate transition from postdoctoral training to a career as an independent investigator.

Comments

Candidates must hold an M.D., D.D.S., D.V.M., D.O., or equivalent degree or nursing degree, have completed clinical training, and have between three (two in the case of nurses) and seven years of postdoctoral experience with some research experience included. In some cases, Ph.D.s with clinical experience, e.g., epidemiology, neuropathology, etc., may be eligible. Candidates are nominated by domestic institutions on the basis of motivation and potential for an academic or research career. Awards are for three- to five-year periods depending on the sponsoring ICD. A minimum of 75 percent effort is required. Allowable costs are up to a $50,000 maximum base salary, with supplementation from nonfederal funds permitted. In addition, $10,000 to $20,000 can be requested for supplies, equipment, travel, etc. Awardees may apply for a FIRST award or a regular research grant. Applications are peer reviewed by institute-managed committees.

Awarding Units and Emphasis Areas

NIA	Geriatric medicine
	Organic brain disease of old age
	Clinical nutrition and aging
	Clinical immunology and aging
	Clinical pharmacology and aging
	Endocrinology and aging
	Maturity onset diabetes and aging
	Dermatology and aging
	Epidemiology and aging
	Musculoskeletal problems and aging
NIAID	Development of basic research skills in the fields of immunology, allergy and immunologic diseases, bacteriology, virology, mycology, parasitology, and epidemiology
NIAMS	Arthritis
	Musculoskeletal disorders
	Skin diseases
NIDDK	Diabetes, endocrine, and metabolic diseases
	Digestive diseases and nutrition
	Kidney, urologic, and blood diseases
NCI	Surgical oncology
	Radiation oncology
	Preventive oncology
	Epidemiology and nutrition
NICHD	Pregnancy and perinatology
	Congenital abnormalities
	Clinical nutrition
	Reproductive biology
	Child and adolescent development
	Mental retardation
	Fertility and infertility
NIEHS	Environmental health/human toxicology

NHLBI	Cardiovascular diseases
	Pulmonary diseases
	Blood diseases and blood-banking sciences
NCNR	Research at any NIH-supported center program, including General Clinical Research Centers, with emphasis on health promotion and disease prevention; acute and chronic illness; and nursing systems
NINDS	Areas of medical science related to neurological disorders and stroke.
NIDCD	Areas of medical science related to deafness and other communication disorders.

Physician Scientist Award (PSA)—Individual (K11)

Description

This is a nonrenewable, phased program designed for clinicians, nominated by domestic institutions, to undertake five years of supervised research training in a fundamental science. Phase I consists of two to three years of study in a basic science laboratory. Phase II is devoted to intensive research activity.

Comments

The purpose is to encourage newly trained clinicians to develop research skills and experience in the basic sciences, e.g., biochemistry, genetics, immunology, etc. Candidates must possess a clinical degree such as M.D., D.D.S., D.V.M., D.O., or equivalent. They should have research potential and a serious intent to pursue research and academic careers. Awardees may apply for a FIRST award or a regular research grant, usually during phase II. A minimum of 75 percent effort is to be devoted to this program. Allowable costs are up to a maximum of $50,000 base salary for full-time, twelve-month activity with supplementation from nonfederal funds permitted; 10 percent of the primary sponsor's salary plus fringe benefits during phase I; and research support of $10,000 to $20,000 per year to cover technical help, supplies, equipment, travel, etc. Applications are peer reviewed by institute-managed committees.

Awarding Units

NCI, NEI, NHLBI, NIA, NIAID, NIAMS, NICHD, NIDDK, NIDR, and NIEHS.

Physician Scientist Award (PSA)—Program (K12)

Description

This is an award that allows institutions to recruit and select candidates locally instead of submitting separate applications for each one. Awards are renewable.

Comments

Program awards are intended to provide support for the development of physician scientists in the same manner as individual awards. Support is limited to two postdoctoral candidates entering phase I per budget period.

Awarding Units

NIA.

Dentist Scientist Award (DSA)—Individual (K15)

Description

This is a nonrenewable, five-year award designed to provide opportunities for dentists, with a strong commitment to oral health research to develop into independent investigators.

Comments

The purpose is the development of competent, dental–clinical scholars with a serious commitment to dental science and who demonstrate a high research potential. Candidates are nominated by domestic institutions. They must have completed a dental degree and devote a minimum of 80 percent time to this research program. The program is to consist of three parts: advanced basic science development, advanced clinical science development, and a supervised research experience. Time commitment for each is not specified; applicants are encouraged to develop integrated, innovative programs taking into account resources available at their institutions. Allowable costs are up to an annual maximum of $50,000 base salary with supplementation from nonfederal funds permitted; up to 5 percent per annum of the salary of the candidate's mentor; and a maximum of $75,000 (not to exceed $20,000 in any one year), for research costs for the five-year period. Applications are peer reviewed by an institute-managed committee.

Awarding Units

NIDR.

Dentist Scientist Award (DSA)—Program (K16)

Description

This award allows institutions to recruit and select candidates locally rather than submitting applications for each one. Awards are renewable.

Comments

Dollar allowances are the same as for the K15 award except for additional allowable costs of up to 10 percent per annum for the salary of a program director. No more than two candidates can be enrolled in the program in a twelve-month budget period.

Awarding Units

NIDR.

TRAINING PROGRAMS: NATIONAL RESEARCH SERVICE AWARDS (NRSA)

Individual Predoctoral Fellowship (F31)

Description

The purpose is to provide predoctoral individuals with supervised research training leading to a Ph.D. or equivalent research degree in specified health and health-related areas.

Comments

Contact awarding units for more information.

Awarding Units

NCI, NIGMS, and NCNR.

Individual Postdoctoral Fellowship (F32)

Description

The purpose is to provide up to three years of postdoctoral research training for basic or clinical scientists to broaden their scientific background and extend their potential in areas that reflect the national need for biomedical and behavioral research.

Comments

Awards are made to individuals. Eligibility requirements are U.S. citizenship or status as a permanent resident, a doctoral degree, and a sponsor well-qualified to supervise the training. Funds may not be used for study leading to professional degrees, e.g., M.D., D.D.S., D.O., etc., or to support residency training. Stipends are based on years of experience. Awardees are subject to NRSA payback provisions; one year of research or teaching, or a combination, is required for each year of support received in excess of twelve months. Most applications are peer reviewed by DRG-managed fellowship panels.

Awarding Units

All NIH awarding units except FIC and NLM.

Senior Postdoctoral Fellowships (F33)

Description

The purpose is to provide up to two years of research opportunities for experienced scientists to make major changes in their research careers either by broadening their scientific backgrounds, acquiring new research capabilities, or enlarging their command of an allied research field.

Comments

Eligibility requirements are a minimum of seven years of relevant postdoctoral research or professional training, U.S. citizenship or status as a permanent resident, and a well-qualified sponsor. NRSA payback provisions apply. Funds may not be used for study leading to professional degrees, e.g., M.D., D.D.S., D.O., etc., or to support residency training. Most applications are peer reviewed by DRG-managed fellowship panels.

Awarding Units

All NIH awarding units except FIC, NLM, and NCRR.

Intramural Individual Postdoctoral Fellowships (F35)

Description

The purpose is to offer basic and clinical biomedical scientists an opportunity to receive full-time research training in the intramural laboratories of several NIH institutes for a period of three years.

Comments

Eligibility requirements are a doctoral degree and U.S. citizenship or permanent resident status. Awardees are subject to NRSA payback provisions. Applications may be received at any time and are usually reviewed semiannually (March and September). The review process includes both an interview with intramural staff and application evaluation by a peer review committee.

Awarding Units

For details, contact:

Deputy Director for Intramural Research
National Institutes of Health
Shannon Bldg., Room 122
Bethesda, MD 20892

Postdoctoral Medical Informatics Fellowship (F37)

Description

The purpose is to provide postdoctoral training in the synthesis, organization, and management of scientific and medical information.

Comments

The training is expected to be interdisciplinary, involving medicine, biotechnology, cognitive sciences, information science, and computer science. For more information, contact NLM.

Awarding Units

NLM.

Institutional National Research Service Awards (T32)

Description

These are awards made to institutions to develop or enhance pre- and postdoctoral research training for individuals interested in preparing for careers in biomedical or behavioral research. Trainees are selected by the institutional program director, who is also responsible for the overall direction of the program.

Comments

Trainees must be U.S. citizens or permanent residents. Funds may not be used to support studies for professional degrees, e.g., M.D., D.D.S., D.O., etc., or residency training. Trainees are subject to NRSA payback provisions. Awards can be made for up to five years and are renewable. Applications are peer reviewed by institute-managed committees.

Awarding Units

All NIH awarding units except for NLM and FIC.

Short-Term Training for Students in Health Professional Schools (T35)

Description

This institutional training program is designed to expose talented students in health professional schools to the possibilities of entering a research career. Research training is for periods of up to three months during the summer or at other appropriate times.

Comments

Awards are for up to five years and are renewable. Domestic schools of medicine, osteopathy, dentistry, veterinary medicine, optometry, pharmacy, and podiatry may apply. The training institution is responsible for selecting trainees who have successfully completed at least one semester. Trainees must be U.S. citizens or permanent residents.

Awarding Units

All NIH awarding units except NCHGR, NCRR, NCNR, FIC, and NLM.

Continuing Education Training Grants (T15)

Description

The purpose is to assist professional schools and other public and nonprofit institutions to establish, expand, or improve programs of continuing professional education.

Comments

Contact staff for more information.

Awarding Units

In FY 1990 NHLBI and in FY 1991 NIA and NCHGR.

Hazardous Waste Worker Health and Safety Training Grant Program (D42)

Description

The purpose is to develop, implement, and evaluate programs to train workers who are or may be engaged in activities related to hazardous waste removal, containment, or emergency response.

Comments

For more information, contact NIEHS.

Awarding Units

NIEHS.

FIC POSTDOCTORAL FELLOWSHIPS

There are a number of fellowship opportunities available to U.S. and foreign health scientists who wish to conduct collaborative research abroad or in this country. The purpose is to promote exchange of research experiences and information in the biomedical sciences. A few of the programs are highlighted below; more details and information about other programs can be obtained by contacting FIC. Also, a *Directory of International Grants and Fellowships in the Health Sciences* can be obtained by writing to:

International Research and Awards Branch
Room 613, Building 38A
FIC, NIH
Bethesda, MD 20892

Programs for U.S. Scientists

Senior International Fellowships (F06)

Description. These fellowships offer opportunities for U.S. biomedical scientists to conduct research in a foreign institution.

Comments. The program is for scientists whose professional stature is well established. Fellowships are awarded for a period of three to twelve months and provide stipend, travel, foreign living allowance, and host institutional allowance.

NIH–French CNRS Program for Scientific Collaboration (F07)

Description. This is an exchange program that allows U.S. scientists to work in French laboratories and French scientists to work in U.S. laboratories.

Comments. The program is a result of an agreement between NIH and the French National Center for Scientific Research (CNRS) that allows qualified scientists to work in either country's laboratories for periods of six months or longer. U.S. scientists must have a doctorate in one of the biomedical sciences or a related field, and recent experience related to any proposed study.

Scholars-in-Residence Program (F15)

Description. The program permits distinguished science leaders and scholars to spend from three to twelve months in residence at NIH.

Comments. For nomination procedures and more information, contact FIC.

Foreign-Supported Fellowships (F20)

Description. These are fellowships to permit U.S. scientists to conduct collaborative research abroad in the specific country providing the funding.

Comments. The maximum period of support is one year; the minimum period varies. Participating countries are Finland, France, Federal Republic of Germany, Ireland, Israel, Japan, Norway, Sweden, Switzerland, and Taiwan.

Program for Foreign Scientists

International Research Fellowships (F05)

Description. These fellowships offer opportunities to foreign scientists in the formative stage of their careers to extend research experiences in U.S. laboratories.

Comments. The purpose of this program is to forge relationships between distinguished scientists in the United States and qualified scientists from other countries. Selections are first made by a nominating committee in a participating country or region. Over fifty countries or regions in the Americas, Africa, Asia and the Far East, Australia, Europe, and New Zealand participate in the program. Fellowships are awarded for a minimum of twelve months and provide stipend, travel, and an institutional allowance.

MISCELLANEOUS GRANT PROGRAMS

Small Grants Program (R03)

Description

The program is designed to provide support, limited in time and dollars, for activities such as pilot projects, testing of new techniques, or feasibility studies of innovative and high-risk research to pave the way for more extended future research efforts. In the case of the NEI, the program is designed to support clinicians with limited research experience, recently trained or less experienced investigators, investigators resuming an interrupted career, investigators changing fields of research, and investigators at minority institutions or in a nonresearch environment. The NHLBI offers support to study readily available clinical trial data bases.

Comments

Awards are nonrenewable. Management of the program varies among institutes. Some restrict awards to certain program areas, others do not; some offer one-year awards, others two-year awards. Most dollar amounts are in the range of $10,000 to $25,000 per year. The NHLBI limit is $50,000 per year for two years. Instructions for preparing applications differ, as do deadline dates. Applications are peer reviewed by institute committees or DRG study sections. Awards cannot be used to supplement other PHS-supported projects. Consultation with program staff is essential to determine requirements of sponsoring institutes.

Awarding Units

NCRR, NIDR, NEI, NIDDK, NCI, NHLBI, NIAID, NCNR, NIDCD, NIA, and NICHD.

Conference Grant (R13)

Description

This is an award that supports international or domestic meetings, conferences, or workshops whose purpose is to coordinate, exchange, and disseminate information related to the program interests of a sponsoring institute.

Comments

Awards are made to organizations eligible to receive NIH research or research training grants, but not to individuals. Normally some cost sharing is expected from the applicant organization. Allowable costs are salaries, consultant services, equipment rental, travel, supplies, conference services, and publications. Indirect costs are not allowed. Applications are evaluated by mail review or by DRG or ICD peer review groups.

Awarding Units

All NIH awarding units sponsor conferences.

Academic Research Enhancement Award (R15)

Description

The award is designed to enhance the research environment of institutions that have not been traditional recipients of NIH research funds. It is a nonrenewable, up to three year award providing up to $75,000 (not more than $35,000 in any one year) for faculty members to initiate or expand research activities in the health sciences.

Comments

The award enables qualified faculty to undertake feasibility studies, pilot studies and other small-scale research projects in order to eventually seek support through the regular NIH grants program. Eligible institutions are those offering baccalaureate or advanced degrees in the sciences related to health. Excluded are those that have received an NIH Biomedical Research Support Grant (BRSG) of $20,000 or more per year for four or more years during the period from FY 1983 through FY 1989. Health professional schools such as schools of medicine, dentistry, nursing, osteopathy, pharmacy, veterinary medicine, public health, allied health, and optometry are eligible. Aside from merit and relevance to NIH programs, funding decisions are based on the institution's past contribution to the undergraduate preparation of doctoral-level health professionals. Applications are peer reviewed by DRG special review committees.

Awarding Units

All awarding units except FIC.

Research Demonstration and Dissemination Projects (R18)

Description

Support is designed to develop, test, and evaluate health service activities, and to foster application of existing knowledge for the control of categorical diseases.

Comments

For more information, contact awarding units.

Awarding Units

NIAID, NIAMS, NCI, NHLBI, and NCNR.

Exploratory/Developmental Grants (R21)

Description

The purpose is to encourage the development of new research activities in categorical program areas.

Comments

Support generally is restricted in time and level of funding. For more information, contact awarding units.

Awarding Units

In FY 1991 NCI, NEI, NIDDK, NICHD, and NCHGR.

Resource-Related Research Projects (R24)

Description

The purpose is to support research projects contributing to improvement of the capability of biomedical research resources.

Comments

For more information, contact NCRR.

Awarding Units

NCRR.

Education Projects (R25)

Description

The purpose is to support a program in one or more of the areas of education, information, training, technical assistance, coordination, or evaluation in a categorical disease area.

Comments

For more information, contact staff.

Awarding Units

In FY 1991 NCI and NCRR.

James A. Shannon Director's Award (R55)

Description

These are awarded for highly meritorious approved R01 and R29 applications that may not receive support because they fall just short of ICD paylines.

Comments

Investigators do not apply for a Shannon Award. New and competing renewal R01 and R29 grant applications with priority scores just beyond ICD paylines would be eligible. This mechanism would provide a discrete, limited award of up to $100,000 total costs for use over a twenty-four-month period with no more than $50,000 to be expended in any one year. Indirect costs are limited to 20 percent and included in the $100,000 total. The NIH intended to make $30 million available for 300 awards with an expected start date of September 1, 1991. Nominations for the Shannon Award would be provided to the OD/NIH by the individual ICD directors. A special panel of NIH scientists will review the ICD nominations and make recommendations to the NIH Director.

Awarding Units

All awarding units except FIC.

Biomedical Research Support Grant (BRSG) (S07)

Description

The BRSG formula grant program provides funds to enhance the research environment of institutions significantly engaged in biomedical and behavioral research supported by the USPHS. These flexible funds, subject to local control, permit grantee institutions to respond quickly to emerging opportunities such as support for pilot studies, research resources, both physical and human, and other research-related needs.

Comments

To receive support, an institution must have received a minimum of $200,000 in PHS research grants during the preceding fiscal year. Grants are awarded to schools of medicine, dentistry, osteopathy, public health, pharmacy, nursing, allied health, optometry, veterinary medicine, and to other academic institutions, hospitals, non-academic research organizations, and state and local health departments.

Awarding Units

NCRR.

Biomedical Research Support Shared Instrumentation Grants (S10)

Description

The program recognizes the need to cope with rapid technological advances in instrumentation and the rapid rate of obsolescence of existing equipment. The objective of the program is to make available, to institutions with a high concentration of PHS-supported investigators, research instruments that can only be justified on a shared-use basis. Awards are limited to instruments/systems that cost at least $100,000. The maximum award is $400,000.

Comments

Eligibility is limited to institutions awarded a BRSG grant. A major user group of three or more investigators should be identified, each with PHS peer-reviewed research support. Awards are for one year and are nonrenewable. Examples of instrumentation supported are NMR systems, electron microscopes, mass spectrometers, protein sequencers/amino acid analyzers, and cell sorters. Applications are reviewed by special peer review groups in DRG.

Awarding Units

NCRR.

NIH Small Instrumentation Grants Program (S15)

Description

The intent of the program is to address the problem of obsolete biomedical research instrumentation costing from $5,000 to $60,000.

Comments

Eligible institutions must have received BRSG support during the preceding fiscal year and have currently active NIH research grants. The amount of the award is based on a percentage of the BRSG award not to exceed $60,000.

Awarding Units

All awarding units except NCRR, NCHGR, and FIC.

TABLE 2A.1. Data on Mechanisms Funded in FY 1991

	Number		Success			Average Total Cost Per Award
	Reviewed	Eligible	Awarded	Rate %	Total Cost	
C06	45	39	8	17.8	21,088,000	2,636,000
D42	3	0	0	0	0	0
F05	153	151	108	70.6	2,841,545	26,311
F06	78	76	39	50.0	1,076,768	27,609
F07	8	8	—	—	—	—
F15	7	7	7	100.0	247,029	35,290
F20	18	17	—	—	—	—
F31	261	247	198	75.9	3,883,284	19,613
F32	1,697	1,624	730	43.0	18,635,056	25,527
F33	44	41	22	50.0	719,358	32,698
F34	9	8	4	44.4	111,000	27,750
F35	4	4	4	100.0	124,600	31,150
F37	4	4	4	100.0	125,400	31,350
G07	34	27	14	41.2	521,745	37,268
G08	17	13	4	23.5	408,573	102,143
G12	12	12	11	91.7	9,161,839	832,894
G20	114	94	46	40.4	10,839,482	235,641
K01	19	18	6	31.6	461,794	76,966
K04	93	87	40	43.0	2,654,510	66,363
K07	91	82	36	39.6	3,706,178	102,949
K08	270	248	143	53.0	10,917,161	76,344
K10	2	1	1	50.0	32,426	32,426
K11	135	131	73	54.1	5,703,424	78,129
K12	2	3	3	100.0	486,939	162,313
K14	4	4	1	25.0	87,703	87,703
K15	9	8	6	66.7	395,362	65,894
K16	1	1	0	0	0	0
M01	59	57	42	71.2	23,654,116	563,193
P01	407	400	207	50.9	159,210,763	769,134
P20	35	31	16	45.7	4,069,481	254,343
P30	160	156	66	41.3	57,741,728	874,875
P40	9	8	3	33.3	1,321,077	440,359
P41	28	28	13	46.4	8,754,326	673,410
P50	85	83	39	45.9	31,275,307	801,931
P51	14	14	13	92.9	7,617,709	585,978
P60	44	37	6	13.6	6,805,259	1,134,210
R01	15,111	14,849	4,190	27.7	809,123,479	193,108
R03	849	727	156	18.4	6,626,395	42,477
R10	6	6	6	100.0	854,465	142,411
R13	295	282	211	71.5	2,787,565	13,211
R15	613	574	139	22.7	13,661,379	98,283
R18	40	30	2	5.0	899,782	449,891
R21	42	41	19	45.2	981,693	51,668
R22	48	48	13	27.1	2,908,543	223,734
R24	38	33	10	26.3	2,308,834	230,883
R25	20	21	19	95.0	2,673,963	140,735
R29	1,455	1,447	454	31.2	44,969,504	99,052
R35	18	21	9	50.0	4,368,176	485,353

(continued)

Table 2A.1. (Continued)

	Number		Success			Average Total Cost Per Award
	Reviewed	Eligible	Awarded	Rate %	Total Cost	
R37	245	253	239	97.6	64,383,739	269,388
R43	1,629	1,090	430	26.4	20,996,056	48,828
R44	292	241	126	43.2	30,942,796	245,578
R55	309	309	309	100.0	15,426,000	49,922
S03	391	391	390	99.7	8,235,000	21,115
S06	56	54	42	75.0	13,564,905	322,974
S07	628	628	628	100.0	22,250,000	35,430
S10	399	375	139	34.8	31,866,000	229,252
S14	5	4	2	40.0	124,676	62,338
S15	593	593	591	99.7	16,189,919	27,394
T14	1	1	1	100.0	75,986	75,986
T15	13	12	7	53.8	384,958	54,994
T32	399	404	253	63.4	41,549,865	164,229
T34	43	42	24	55.8	1,810,368	75,432
T35	40	38	26	65.0	823,633	31,678
T36	1	1	1	100.0	84,286	84,286
U01	389	355	125	32.1	54,123,353	432,987
U09	8	8	8	100.0	5,963,000	745,375
U10	214	145	77	36.0	21,566,320	280,082
U42	1	1	1	100.0	554,213	554,213
U54	4	4	4	100.0	3,074,778	768,695

Totals for all mechanisms:

Applications reviewed	28,170
Applications recommended	26,614
Carryovers	183
Eligible for award	26,797
Awarded	10,564
Total costs awarded	1,640,825,571 (competing grant awards)
Percent of budget for competing grant awards	25.9
Percent of budget for non-competing awards	74.1

*Source: ISB, DRG

Included in the eligible category are 183 carryovers from the previous fiscal year. They are dispersed over many mechanisms and not separately identified.

Data for mechanisms for underrepresented minorities are included. These mechanisms are described separately in Appendix 3.

Research Facilities Construction Grants (C06)

Description

The purpose is to provide matching funds for construction or major remodeling to create new research facilities.

Comments

Contact awarding units for more information.

Awarding Units

In FY 1991 NCI, NEI, and NHLBI.

Resources Improvement Grant (G07)

Description

This is a non-renewable grant to establish a library or expand or improve present libraries that have inadequate resources relative to their needs and user population.

Comments

Contact NLM for more information.

Awarding Units

NLM.

Resources Project Grant (G08)

Description

This is an award to medical libraries that meet minimal standards and propose plans for the improvement of services as opposed to the acquisition of basic resources.

Comments

Contact NLM for more information.

Awarding Units

NLM.

Grants for Repair, Renovation, and Modernization of Existing Research Facilities (G20)

Description

The purpose is to provide funds for major repair, renovation, and modernization of existing research facilities.

Comments

Facilities may include clinical, animal, and other related research facilities. For more information, contact NCRR.

Awarding Units

NCRR.

COOPERATIVE AGREEMENTS

Research Project (Cooperative Agreement) (U01)

Description

This is the same type of award as an R01 except for required cooperative working arrangement with NIH staff.

Comments

Applications are solicited via RFAs.

Awarding Units

In FY 1991, NIA, NIAID, NCI, NIDCD, NIDDK, NICHD, and NHLBI.

Cooperative Clinical Research (Cooperative Agreement) (U10)

Description

Awards to support clinical trials of various methods of therapy or prevention usually conducted under established protocols.

Comments

Applications usually solicited via RFAs.

Awarding Units

In FY 1991, NCI, NEI, and NICHD.

Resource-Related Research Projects (Cooperative Agreements) (U24)

Description

Same as R24 except for cooperative arrangement with NCRR staff.

Comments

For more information, contact NCRR staff.

Awarding Units

NCRR.

Animal Resource (Cooperative Agreement) (U42)

Description

Same as P40 except for cooperative arrangement with NCRR staff.

Comments

For more information, contact NCRR staff.

Awarding Units

NCRR.

Appendix 3

Extramural Support Mechanisms for Underrepresented Minorities

MINORITY ACCESS TO RESEARCH CAREERS (MARC) PROGRAM

This is a multifaceted program designed to help institutions with substantial minority enrollments to strengthen science curricula and research opportunities and to increase research capabilities of minority scientists. Several types of awards are available. The program is managed by the NIGMS.

MARC Honors Undergraduate Research Training Program (T34)

Description

The program has three objectives: (1) to increase the number of well-prepared minority students who can compete successfully for entry into graduate programs leading to a Ph.D.; (2) to aid the development of a strong biological sciences curriculum; and (3) to strengthen biomedical and behavioral research training programs.

Comments

Eligible institutions are two- and four-year colleges and universities with a significant proportion, usually higher than 50 percent, of minority students as well as Indian tribes with recognized governing bodies. In addition to institutions located in the United States, those in Puerto Rico, the Virgin Islands, the Canal Zone, Guam, American Samoa, or the Trust Territory of the Pacific Islands are eligible.

Stipends and tuition fees are provided for junior- and senior-level honor students and for equipment, supplies, and trainee travel. Maximum support period is five years.

MARC Predoctoral Fellowship (F31)

Description

The award provides support for research training leading to the Ph.D. for graduates of the MARC Honors Undergraduate Research Training Program.

Comments

Support is not available for individuals enrolled in medical or other professional schools. An annual stipend is included as well as funds for the sponsoring institution for tuition, supplies, trainee travel, and related expenses.

MARC Faculty Fellowship (F34)

Description

The award offers opportunities for additional research training for faculty members at institutions eligible for MARC support.

Comments

Faculty members can undertake predoctoral or postdoctoral research training for periods up to three years. At completion of training, fellows are expected to return to their institutions to engage in research and teaching.

MARC Visiting Scientist Award (F36)

Description

The award enables qualifying institutions to support visiting scientists for the benefit of students and faculty.

Comments

Visiting scientists should be recognized scientist–scholars in biomedical disciplines or clinical areas. Support is for periods of three to twelve months with the stipend dependent on current salary as well as a travel allowance.

MINORITY BIOMEDICAL RESEARCH SUPPORT (MBRS) PROGRAM (S06)

Description

The purpose of the program is to strengthen the capability of minority institutions (1) to provide health career opportunities for students and (2) to conduct research in the health sciences.

Comments

Eligible institutions are two- and four-year colleges and universities with a significant proportion, usually higher than 50 percent, of minority students. Indian tribes with recognized governing bodies are included. In addition to institutions located in the United States, those in Puerto Rico, the Virgin Islands, the Canal Zone, Guam, American Samoa, or the Trust Territory of the Pacific Islands are eligible.

There are four types of awards:

1. The traditional type of MBRS grant to enrich the institutional environment and provide the resources for a broad spectrum of faculty and student research activities.
2. The MBRS Undergraduate grant to support one or more of the following for periods up to three years: (a) biomedical enrichment activities such as seminars, travel to scientific meetings, workshops, and off-campus research activities during the summer for faculty and students; (b) pilot projects; and (c) research projects.
3. The MBRS Thematic Project grant is aimed at institutions with Ph.D. programs and health professional schools. Only one application can be submitted per eligible institution. The purpose is to assist developing graduate programs and to foster interdepartmental collaboration around specific research themes or disciplines. The usual research costs are allowable except for student support, which should be obtained from other MBRS funds. Support for no less than three nor more than five subprojects will be provided with a $300,000 limit per year for up to four years.
4. The MBRS supplemental grant for shared instrumentation. Please see BRSG (S10) award in Appendix 2.

Awarding Units

NIGMS.

RESEARCH CENTERS IN MINORITY INSTITUTIONS (RCMI) PROGRAM (G12)

Description

The purpose is to establish research centers in those predominantly minority institutions that offer doctoral degrees in the health professions or the health-related sciences. The program is designed to provide grants of up to $1 million per year, for five years, to help eligible institutions enrich their research environments through selected improvements in their human and physical resources.

Comments

An institution must have more than 50 percent minority enrollment, award an M.D., D.D.S., D.V.M., or other doctoral degrees in the health professions, or a Ph.D. in the sciences related to health. Funds can be used to support central resources such as animal facilities, instrument and machine shops; purchase and installation of equipment; alterations and renovations; salaries of key research and research-support personnel; consultant costs; supplies; travel; library support; and patient costs. Support is intended to complement ongoing and planned research activities funded by MBRS and MARC programs, traditional NIH and ADAMHA research grants, and NRSA awards in the biomedical and behavioral sciences.

Awarding Units

NCRR.

MINORITY HIGH SCHOOL STUDENT RESEARCH APPRENTICE PROGRAM (S03)

Description

The program is designed to stimulate interest among minority high school students in scientific careers.

Comments

To be eligible, an institution must have been the recipient of either a BRSG or MBRS award during the last federal fiscal year. Support of $1,500 per apprentice position will be provided for students enrolled in a high school during an academic year coinciding with the award. Funds are intended for hourly salaries and supplies. Program directors are responsible for recruitment, selection, and assignment of students to interested investigators conducting biomedical research. Applications are due December 1 and need only consist of a one-page letter stating the number of positions requested and applicable information on the Form 398 face page.

Awarding Units

NCRR.

NHLBI MINORITY SUMMER PROGRAM IN PULMONARY RESEARCH (T35S)

Description

The program is intended to encourage qualified minority faculty and graduate students to develop interests in pulmonary research.

Comments

Trainees must participate in a program at an established pulmonary training center. The center must have a demonstrated research capability and provide assurance of cooperation with one or more minority institutions. Stipends for both faculty members and graduate students are provided, as well as trainee-related costs.

Awarding Unit

NHLBI.

NHLBI MINORITY INSTITUTIONAL RESEARCH TRAINING PROGRAM (T32M)

Description

Awards are offered in cardiovascular, pulmonary, and hematologic research to minority schools to train graduate students and to stimulate research, prevention, control, and education efforts in these areas.

Comments

The minority institution must collaborate with a research center that has strong, well-established cardiovascular, pulmonary, or hematologic research and research training programs. The Program Director is responsible for selection and appointment of trainees who must be at the postbaccalaureate level. Stipend levels and related support are similar to those for NRSA predoctoral trainees.

Awarding Units

NHLBI.

NHLBI MINORITY SCHOOL FACULTY DEVELOPMENT AWARD (K14)

Description

The award is intended to encourage the development of faculty investigators at minority schools in areas relevant to cardiovascular, pulmonary, and hematologic diseases and resources.

Comments

Candidates must have a doctoral degree or equivalent in a biomedical science and have the potential to benefit from additional training. Each is to work with an accomplished mentor at a nearby research center (within 100 miles). Salary support up to a maximum of $50,000 per year plus fringe benefits can be requested in addition to $20,000 per year in other research costs.

Awarding Units

NHLBI.

NIH EXTRAMURAL ASSOCIATES PROGRAM

Description

This program allows faculty or individuals in key administrative posts at minority institutions to receive a maximum of one year of administrative training at the NIH.

Comments

The program offers intensive administrative training under the supervision of the NIH extramural staff. Support is arranged through the Intergovernmental Personnel Act. Since its inception in 1978, more than fifty individuals have participated in this program. For more information, contact:

> **Extramural Associates Program**
> **Building 31, Room 5B38**
> **NIH,**
> **Bethesda, MD 20892**
> **(301) 496–9728**

Awarding Units

Office of Director, NIH.

There are several support mechanisms previously described in Appendix 2 which may be of particular interest. These are identified in Table 3A.1. Additionally, the following opportunities can be explored:

TABLE 3A.1. Summary of Programs of Interest of Underrepresented Minorities

Target Group	Sponsor
High School Students	
Research Apprenticeship Program for Minority High School Students (S03)	NCRR
Undergraduate Students	
Marc Honors Undergraduate Research Training Program (T34)	NIGMS
Minority Biomedical Research Support Program (S06)	NIGMS
Research Supplements for Minority Undergraduate Students (see Chapter 4)	All NIH
Postbaccalaureate Students	
NHLBI Minority Summer Program in Pulmonary Research (T35S)	NHLBI
Minority Biomedical Research Support Program (S06)	NIGMS
MARC Predoctoral Fellowship Award (F31)	NIGMS
Research Supplements for Minority Graduate Research Assistants (see Chapter 4)	All NIH
NHLBI Minority Institutional Research Training Program (T32M)	NHLBI
Other NIH Programs of Special Interest	
NRSA for Institutional Training (T32)	All NIH
Short-term Training for Students in Health Professional Schools (T35)	All NIH
NRSA Individual Predoctoral Fellowships (F31)	NCNR
Postdoctoral Students	
Minority Biomedical Research Support Program (S06)	NIGMS
Other NIH Programs of Special Interest	
NRSA for Institutional Training (T32)	All NIH
NRSA Individual Postdoctoral Fellowships (F32)	All NIH
NIH Staff Fellowships (NIH Intramural Program)	
NIH Medical Staff Fellowship Program (NIH Intramural Program)	
Postdoctoral/Faculty	
Minority Biomedical Research Support Program (S06)	NIGMS
MARC Faculty Fellowship (F34)	NIGMS
MARC Visiting Scientist Award (F36)	NIGMS
Minority School Faculty Development Award (K14)	NHLBI
NHLBI Minority Summer Program in Pulmonary Research (T35S)	NHLBI
Research Supplements for Minority Investigators (see Chapter 4)	All NIH
NIH Extramural Associate Program	OD/NIH
Other NIH Programs of Special Interest	
NRSA Senior Fellowships (F33)	*
Senior International Fellowships (F06)	*
Research Career Development Award (K04)	*
Academic/Teacher Award (K07)	*
Clinical Investigator Award (K08)	*
Physician Scientist Award (K11)	*
FIRST Award (R29)	*
Small Grants Program (R03)	*
Grants Associate Program	OD/NIH

(*continued*)

TABLE 3A.1. (*Continued*)

Target Group	Sponsor
Institutional Awards	
Minority Biomedical Research Support Program (S06)	NIGMS
Research Centers in Minority Institutions (G12)	NCRR
Other NIH Programs of Special Interest	
Academic Research Enhancement Award (R15)	All NIH

*See Appendix 2.

NIH Staff Fellowships

The program enables scientists with M.D., D.D.S., Ph.D., or equivalent degrees, to work in NIH intramural laboratories. For more information, contact:

Office of Special Programs
Room 2N230, Clinical Center
NIH
Bethesda, MD 20892
(301) 496–2427

NIH Clinical Associate Program

The program enables clinicians (M.D., D.D.S., or equivalent degree) to acquire research training in NIH intramural laboratories. For more information, contact:

NIH Clinical Associates Program
Room 2N226, Clinical Center
Bethesda, MD 20892
(301) 496–2427

Grants Associate Program

The program provides a year of intensive, administrative experience in the NIH extramural programs. A doctorate or equivalent degree in a discipline related to biomedical or behavioral sciences is required. Those selected become full-time federal employees. For more information, contact:

NIH Grants Associate Program
Office of Extramural Research
Room 5B-32, Building 31
Bethesda, MD 20892
(301) 496–1736

Appendix 4

DRG Study Section Assignment Areas

MECHANISMS REVIEWED

- Research Project Grant (R01)
- Academic Research Enhancement Award (R15)
- U.S.–Japan Cooperative Medical Science Program (R22)
- First Independent Research Support and Transition Award (R29)
- Small Business Innovation Research Awards (R43, R44)
- Fogarty International Center Fellowships (F05, F06)
- Individual Postdoctoral Fellowship (F32)
- Senior Fellowship (F33)
- Research Career Development Award (K04)
- Biomedical Research Support Shared Instrumentation Grant (S10)
- Short-term Training Award (T35)
- Conference Grant (R13) (occasionally)
- Program Project Grant (P01) (occasionally)

BEHAVIORAL AND NEUROSCIENCES REVIEW SECTION

Behavioral Medicine (BEM)

Behavioral factors as causes of disease or influences on health maintenance; interventions to change health and health behaviors; behavioral sequelae of disease or the treatment for disease.

Behavioral and Neurosciences 1 (BNS-1)

This panel reviews fellowship applications in the areas of: neurology; neuroanatomy; developmental neurobiology, neurochemistry; neurophysiology; neuropsychology; neuropharmacology.

Behavioral and Neurosciences 2 (BNS-2)

This panel reviews fellowship applications in the areas of: experimental, comparative, social, behavioral, developmental, biopsychological, gerontological, behavioral medicine; sociology; demography; population studies; language development; linguistics; audiology.

Bio-Psychology (BPO)

Conditioning and learning; sensory functions; comparative studies of behavior; neuroanatomy, neurophysiology, neurochemistry and neuropharmacology as related to behavior in animals or humans; developmental neurobiology; hormones and behavior.

Sensory Disorders and Language (CMS)

Voice and voice mechanisms; speech and language development; neurological disorders in language and speech; taste, smell and chemical communication; tactile and somatic sensation; intersensory comparisons.

Hearing Research (HAR)

Otorhinology; otologic physiology; audiology; vestibular system; head and neck surgery; development and plasticity in the auditory and vestibular systems.

Human Development and Aging 1 (HUD-1)

Normal infant development; normal child development; normal adolescent and early adult development; normal cognitive development; social, emotional, and personality development; family structure and processes; normal language development; reading; theory development (developmental, personality, social, cognitive domains); behavior genetics; nutrition (nutrition and development, nutrition and behavior).

Human Development and Aging 2 (HUD-2)

Well-being and adjustment in aging; health and aging; environmental psychology and aging; living arrangements; behavioral factors in long-term care and institutionalization; cross-cultural and ethnic studies of aging; social psychology of the aging; life-span developmental studies; senile dementia and Alzheimer's disease (behavioral and neuropsychological measures); cognitive psychology and aging; memory and learning in aging; human factors and training in adult and older

populations; functional ability and intelligence; psychology and sociology of inter-
generational relations.

Human Development and Aging 3 (HUD-3)

Consequences of pregnancy and birth; developmental consequences of neurological
diseases, physiological disorders, and specific genetic disorders; problems of infan-
cy; dysfunctional child development; dysfunctional adolescent development and
disorders of adolescence; disorders in language acquisition; problems of social and
personality development; problems of perceptual and cognitive development; learning disabilities; developmental effects of prenatal and postnatal exposure to environmental toxins, alcohol, and drugs; mental retardation; individual, family, and community coping and adjustment of the retarded child, adolescent, and adult;
intervention research; applied analysis of behavior.

Neurology A (NEUA)

Clinical neurology; neuroanatomy (basic studies of the CNS, in neurological diseases and after injury as in stroke, head injury, epilepsy); neurochemistry; neurophysiology (basic and clinical studies in the CNS, electrophysiology of epilepsy
and other diseases, EEG, evoked potentials, event-related potentials, physiology of
movement control systems); neurosurgery (trauma in the CNS); brain imaging.

Neurology B 1 (NEUB-1)

Neurophysiology (basic aspects, especially studies of synaptic and motor system
physiology); neuroanatomy (basic ultrastructural studies); preclinical neurology;
CNS development and regeneration; neurochemistry ; neuropathology (animal models for experimental conditions); neurosurgery (experimental, posttraumatic, or
postsurgical nervous system regeneration).

Neurology B 2 (NEUB-2)

Nervous system development (morphological and neurophysiological analyses of
structure–function relationships); neuroanatomy (developmental and comparative);
neurophysiology (in vivo and in vitro studies of the developing nervous system);
neuropsychology; autonomic functions.

Neurological Sciences 1 (NLS-1)

Neural cell biology; intermediary metabolism (classes of compounds involved in
neural structure and function); cellular components (CNS or peripheral nervous

system); biochemical characterization (nervous tissue, cells, cellular organelles, and macromolecules of nervous system origin); biochemical and biophysical events in neurotransmission.

Neurological Sciences 2 (NLS-2)

Neurotransmitter receptors (biochemical characterization, receptor regulation); pain mechanisms; neurotransmitter function; basic science studies in the neurological diseases and aging (animal models and in vitro studies).

Social Sciences and Population (SSP)

Fertility (antecedents and consequences, trends, measurement, and prediction as affected by marriage, divorce, child spacing, status of women); migration, immigration and population redistribution; mortality, morbidity, functioning and disability; family planning; infertility; population size, composition, and structure; policy studies; household and family structure; employment and retirement.

Visual Sciences A (VISA)

Clinical ophthalmic research (congenital and developmental abnormalities, inflammatory and infectious diseases, heredofamilial and degenerative, tumors, injury and trauma, etc.); experimental ophthalmic research (development and use of diagnostic and therapeutic devices and procedures); fundamental ophthalmic research (anatomy, physiology, biochemistry, physical chemistry, immunochemistry); epidemiology of eye disease.

Visual Sciences B (VISB)

Psychophysical studies of the visual sense (visual constancies, binocular space sense, physiological optics of simple and compound eyes, control mechanisms of the eye); structure and function of the higher visual pathways (histological, electrophysiological, and biochemical techniques for a better understanding of color vision, stereopsis, and pattern recognition); theoretical studies of the above; instrumentation, e.g., mobility devices for the blind at the developmental stage.

Visual Sciences C (VISC)

Anatomical, physiological, biochemical and biophysical studies of the retina; mechanisms of vision and visual disorders; clinical and fundamental research on the etiology, prevention, diagnosis, and treatment of retinal and choroidal diseases; visual pigments (biochemical and biological functions in phototransduction); models of neural interconnections in the retina; instrumentation and computer technology in vision research related to the retina; genetic and molecular biological studies of the retina.

BIOLOGICAL SCIENCES REVIEW SECTION

Biological Sciences 1 (BIOL-1)

This panel reviews fellowship applications in the areas of: genetics of prokaryotic and eukaryotic organisms (gene expression, genetic regulation, transcription, gene transfer).

Biological Sciences 2 (BIOL-2)

This panel reviews fellowship application in the areas of: cellular and molecular biological aspects of all eukaryotic systems except fungi, plants, and yeast (synthesis, structure, and composition of biological macromolecular and related interactions; molecular aspects of cells; extracellular matrix; gene organization and biochemical basis for gene expression, genetic regulation and transcription in normal and pathological states; mechanism of hormonal action at molecular level; biochemistry of nucleic acid and protein synthesis; control of cell growth and proliferation; structure of microtubules, microfilaments, and intermediate filaments; cellular molecular development; molecular neurogenetics).

Biological Sciences 3 (BIOL-3)

This panel reviews fellowship applications in the areas of: cellular and molecular biological aspects of prokaryotes, yeast, fungi, parasites, plants (cellular organization, development, and interaction between cells; cellular and microbial physiology; basic biology of pathogenic organisms).

Bacteriology and Mycology 1 (BM-1)

Host–parasite relationships; pathogenesis (leprosy, tuberculosis, syphilis, chlamydial infections); etiology (bacterial diseases); basic biology of bacterial disease agents.

Bacteriology and Mycology 2 (BM-2)

Host–parasite relationships; pathogenesis (diseases caused by *Mycoplasma* and *Legionella*); etiology (fungal and bacterial diseases); diagnostic procedures and vaccine preparation; environmental conditions in relation to bacterial and fungal agents and the host; food microbiology; basic biology of disease agents.

Cellular Biology and Physiology 1 (CBY-1)

Cell organization; structure and function of plasma membranes; structural and functional aspects of cell motility; endocytosis and exocytosis; differentiation and embryogenesis.

Cellular Biology and Physiology 2 (CBY-2)

Growth and phenotypic expression of differentiated functions of cells in vitro; regulation of the cell cycle; structure and function of cell membranes; regulation of active transport systems.

Molecular Cytology (CTY)

Chromatin structure and function; biochemistry of cells and tissues and of cellular organelles and components; fine structure of cells; membrane and cell surface biochemistry; control of cellular growth and proliferation; nonmuscle motility; plant molecular biology.

Genetics (GEN)

Genetics; molecular and biochemical genetics; developmental genetics; cytogenetics; mutagenesis; transmission genetics; population and quantitative genetics.

Genome (GNM)

Genetic mapping; physical mapping; DNA sequencing; development of new biophysical and analytical chemistry methodologies directed toward the genome project; data management and analysis.

International and Cooperative Projects (ICP)

This panel reviews fellowship applications for international awards mainly supported by or processed through the Fogarty International Center, but also supported by the various ICDs involving the biological, biomedical, physiological, clinical, behavioral, and neurological sciences.

Microbial Physiology and Genetics 1 (MBC-1)

Functional studies (e.g., cell surface phenomena, growth, metabolism, and regulation of these processes); microbial structure and chemical studies; organisms; methodologies (biochemistry, biophysics, genetics).

Microbial Physiology and Genetics 2 (MBC-2)

Microbial DNA replication, recombination, and transfer; DNA mutagenesis and repair; plasmid DNA replication, transfer, plasmid incompatibility, and plasmid immunity; mechanisms of bacteriophage DNA replication, mechanisms of lysogeny and transduction; transformation, transposition, and conjugation in DNA transfer between bacteria; gene cloning; transcription and translation of microbial DNA; ribosomal RNA synthesis; transfer RNA synthesis and RNA processing.

Molecular Biology (MBY)

DNA synthesis and control of DNA replication (eukaryotic systems); gene organization and function of the genome; transcription mechanisms including enzymology; molecular determinants in regulation of translation and developmental processes; mitochondrial biogenesis and mitochondrial membranes.

Mammalian Genetics (MGN)

Biochemical genetics; medical genetics; molecular genetics; somatic cell genetics; immunogenetics (molecular or with disease associations); cytogenetics; population genetics; developmental genetics (warm-blooded species); behavioral genetics; mutagenesis.

Neurology C (NEUC)

Neurogenetics; general biochemical neuropathology (immune system as the cause of the pathology); neural development and differentiation (biochemical and macromolecular aspects of normal and abnormal embryonic neural determination and differentiation); neurological–immunological interactions (nervous system-oriented protocols); neuroimmunopathology (brain lesions of immunological origin); growth factors and oncogenes with regard to normal and abnormal differentiation and function of the nervous system.

Tropical Medicine and Parasitology (TMP)

Biomedical (diagnosis, prophylaxis, and chemotherapy, vaccine development, epidemiology, etc.); biochemistry (metabolic pathways, mechanism of vector control by bacterial toxins, membrane transport); genetics (control of vectors, genetic control of metabolic systems); host-parasite relationships; immunoparasitology; vectors (mollusks/arthropods); hormones (endocrinology of invertebrates).

BIOMEDICAL SCIENCES REVIEW SECTION

Molecular and Cellular Biophysics (BBCA)
Physical chemistry of biological macromolecules; spectroscopy; protein folding and nucleic acid conformations; theoretical and computational chemistry; thermodynamics; kinetics; photophysics and photochemistry.

Biophysical Chemistry (BBCB)

Physical chemistry of biological macromolecules; spectroscopy; membranes (structure and physical chemistry); physical chemical instrumentation.

Biochemistry (BIO)

Regulation (general enzymology); protein structure and function; cyclic nucleotides; nucleic acids.

Biomedical Sciences (BIOM)

This panel reviews fellowship applications in the areas of: enzymology; bioenergetics; metabolic pathways; biosynthesis; chemical structure of cells and tissues; radiation biology and therapy; molecular biophysics; chemical and physical properties and structure of macromolecules; medicinal chemistry; organic synthesis and methodology; natural products; chemical cellular pathology; chemical carcinogenesis.

Metallobiochemistry (BMT)

Bioinorganic chemistry; metal-containing natural products; organometalloid chemistry; analytical methods; clinical chemistry.

Bio-Organic and Natural Products Chemistry (BNP)

Bio-organic chemistry (chemical evolutionary studies of natural products, design and synthesis of enzyme substrates, antagonists and inhibitors); natural products (isolation, separation, and structure determination); medicinal and pharmaceutical chemistry.

Chemical Pathology (CPA)

Induction of cellular and subcellular lesions; induction of tumors by chemical and physical means; synthesis of carcinogenic and toxic substances; in vitro carcinogenesis; spectroscopic techniques.

Medical Biochemistry (MEDB)

Inborn errors of metabolism (cystinosis, glycinemia, maple syrup urine disease, PKU, etc.); biochemistry of other diseases and syndromes (cystic fibrosis, Reye's syndrome, etc.); disease mechanisms (enzyme inhibitors in body fluids and tissues during disease states); diagnostic biochemistry; animal models; role of prostaglandins in inflammatory responses.

Medicinal Chemistry (MCHA)

Medicinal and pharmaceutical chemistry (total synthesis or synthetic methodology, routine synthesis with substantial measures of in vivo or in vitro pharmacological evaluation); structure determined by synthesis or degradation; development of synthetic organic or organometallic methodology; chemical dynamics.

Metabolism (MET)

Metabolism of carbohydrates (insulin, glucagon, somatastatin, glycogenesis, gluconeogenesis, glycolysis, diabetes mellitus); metabolism of amino acids and proteins (regulation of metabolism and metabolic control of pathways); metabolism of lipids (lipoproteins, cholesterol, chylomicrons, lipogenesis regulation of adipose tissue metabolism, hyperlipidemias, atherogenesis, obesity).

Physical Biochemistry (PB)

Electron transport (bioenergetics, oxidative phosphorylation, energy transfer); enzyme mechanisms (enzyme kinetics, metal cofactors and enzyme action, flavoproteins); protein structure (sequencing to determine primary structure); membranes (synthetic vesicles and reconstitution in the study of bacterial and mammalian transport, membranes and the interaction of phospholipids, and proteins in membranes).

Pathobiochemistry (PBC)

Connective tissue and extracellular matrix biochemistry; protein biochemistry (characterization, biosynthesis, degradation, structure–function relations of proteins in normal and disease states); enzymology (disease related); nucleic acid biochemistry (genetic regulatory mechanisms); membrane biochemistry (structure–function and biosynthesis in normal and disease states, biochemistry of nonsensory cell surface receptors); biochemistry of aging; biochemistry of disease (genetic and pulmonary).

Physiological Chemistry (PC)

Protein chemistry (purification, structure–function relationships); protein biosynthesis; nucleic acid chemistry (biosynthesis of DNA and RNA and enzymes involved); enzymes (regulation and mechanisms); carbohydrate biochemistry, lipids; biomembrane structure and function (isolation and characterization); hormones (structure, membrane receptor reactions).

Radiation (RAD)

Therapeutic radiology; therapeutic hyperthermia; radiation (medical) physics; radiation biology; radiation biophysics and biochemistry (interaction of radiation in vivo and in vitro).

CLINICAL SCIENCES REVIEW SECTION

Clinical Sciences 1 (CLIN-1)

This panel reviews fellowship applications in the areas of: gastroenterology; hematology; rheumatology; hepatology; dermatology; nutrition; oncology (GI tract and blood); orthopedics (bone calcification and histopathology of bone disease).

Clinical Sciences 2 (CLIN-2)

This panel reviews fellowship applications in the areas of: circulation; hypertension; neural control of cardiovascular system; pulmonary physiology; exercise and muscle physiology; renin-angiotensin; surgery; diagnostic radiology and imaging.

Cardiovascular and Pulmonary (CVA)

Cardiac function; maturation and aging of the heart; control of cardiac function; metabolic studies; coronary circulation; in vitro studies of cardiac tissue; pathology (morphology and ultrastructure of the heart when correlated with physiologic or biochemical findings); cardiopulmonary system (interactions of pulmonary and cardiac functions).

Cardiovascular and Renal (CVB)

Clinical cardiology; basic studies of myocardial function; electrophysiology and electrocardiology; circulation; blood pressure (kallikrein, kinin, and bradykinin systems; cardiac dynamics and function related to hypertension).

Experimental Cardiovascular Sciences (ECS)

Blood flow studies; vascular smooth muscle; neural control of the circulation and kidneys; blood pressure, e.g., anti-hypertensive drugs; studies of the heart (cardiac dysfunction related to peripheral vascular disease).

General Medicine A 1 (GMA-1)

Rheumatic disease–connective tissue disease; metabolic diseases (diseases of mineral metabolism, diseases of osteoid tissue, cystic fibrosis, hyperuricemia, gout); dermatology.

General Medicine A 2 (GMA-2)

Gastroenterology; gastrointestinal physiology; gastrointestinal metabolism; gastroenteric endocrinology; neurogastroenterology; gastrointestinal pharmacology; clinical nutrition (related to gastroenterology).

Hematology 1 (HEM-1)

General hematology; blood formation; hemoglobin; coagulation, anticoagulants, fibrinolysis; metabolism of red and white blood cells; immunohematology, blood groups, transfusion; anemia.

Hematology 2 (HEM-2)

The same as HEM-1.

Metabolic Pathology (MEP)

Role of nutrients in the induction of cellular and subcellular lesions and in tumorigenesis by physical and chemical means; role of nutrients in the prevention of tumorigenesis; role of nutrition or specific nutrients in experimental and clinical cancer and other disease conditions, e.g., hepatic disease, gastrointestinal disease; cellular mechanisms by which nutrients modulate tumorigenesis.

Nutrition (NTN)

Requirements of normal living organisms for protein, fat, carbohydrate, vitamins, and trace minerals; nutritional practices in obesity, malnutrition, pregnancy, childhood, the aged; alteration of biochemical and physiological lesions by dietary practice (diabetes, atherosclerosis, etc.); effects of nutrition or specific nutrients on resistance to disease; biochemical and physiological effects of malnutrition; methods of evaluating the nutritive status of humans; application of techniques for measuring body composition; nutritive value of raw and processed foods and factors affecting them.

Nursing Research (NURS)

Health promotion and disease prevention (studies of the general health of the population and to decrease the vulnerability of individuals and families to illness or disability); acute and chronic illness (biomedical, behavioral, and environmental factors that contribute to the cause, prevalence, amelioration, and remediation of illness and disability); nursing systems (the environment in which nursing care is delivered, promising approaches to nursing management, and nursing care delivery); ethics (related to patient care and patient care research).

Orthopedics and Musculoskeletal (ORTH)

Orthopedics; bone and cartilage metabolism (calcification of bone, bone cell culture, radiographic diagnosis of bone disease, histopathology of bone disease, osteoporosis, and osteogenesis imperfecta); bioengineering (biomechanics of the skeleton and joints); biomaterials; sports medicine; neurophysiology (motor control of limb movement); muscle, ligament, and tendon physiology (biomechanics and surgery); osteopathy and chiropractic.

Respiratory and Applied Physiology (RAP)

Respiration (respiratory mechanics, ventilation–perfusion, neural and chemical control of breathing, effect of high altitude and hyperbaric pressure, dysfunction during sleep, respiratory muscle function and fatigue, bioengineering of the lung and pulmonary vasculature, cardiopulmonary interactions); exercise/work physiology; environmental physiology (physiological responses to extremes of temperature, pressure, and humidity); muscle (physiology and pathophysiology related to exercise and work, muscle metabolism, histology, and histochemistry, molecular biology of skeletal muscle).

Diagnostic Radiology (RNM)

Diagnostic X rays (new and improved instrumentation and techniques for radiography, contrast media, digital subtraction angiography, fluoroscopy, computerized tomography); nuclear medicine (production and in vivo distribution of radiopharmaceuticals); ultrasound (production and detection of ultrasound for diagnosis); magnetic resonance imaging (MRI or NMR); image processing and evaluation.

Surgery, Anesthesiology, and Trauma (SAT)

Cardiac, vascular, and pulmonary disease and abnormalities (diagnosis, surgical care or treatment, evaluation of results); anesthesiology (experimental or clinical); shock, trauma, and burns; transplantation, grafting, and reconstruction (transplantation of whole organs or tissue mass, experimentally or clinically); urology.

Surgery and Bioengineering (SB)

Cardiac, vascular, and pulmonary diseases and abnormalities (surgical diagnosis, care, treatment, or evaluation); bioengineering, biomaterials, bioinstrumentation, and biomathematics (excludes orthopedics); surgical gastroenterology.

IMMUNOLOGY, VIROLOGY AND PATHOLOGY
REVIEW SECTION

Allergy and Immunology (ALY)

Immunochemistry (molecular and structural study of components of immunocompetent cell activity); immunogenetics (biochemistry of genetic control of antibody synthesis); immunodeficiency states (biochemical assessment of immunologic states in health and disease, lymphokines, cytokines); general immune response (biochemical and molecular aspects).

AIDS and Related Research 1 (ARRA)

Humoral antibody response in AIDS; cellular immune response (role of immunocompetent cells in HIV infection and in immune deficiency); immune deficiency state (the function of immunologic mediators in establishing the immune deficiency state and immunologic factors in prenatal HIV infection); immunologic characterization of cellular and viral components; animal model systems.

AIDS and Related Research 2 (ARRB)

Geographic and social distribution of the infection or disease and of related factors (spread of HIV infection in designated risk groups); horizontal and vertical transmission of the infection; identification of the biologic, genetic, and psychosocial risk factors; development and improvement of research designs and methodologies; development and application of mathematical and statistical models of the status and progression of the infection/disease.

AIDS and Related Research 3 (ARRC)

Molecular biological studies of HIV and related viruses; genetic studies (interactions between HIV and other viruses, regulation of gene function, isolation of mutants, DNA repair, gene mapping and sequencing); pathogenesis (disease development); biochemistry of viral infection; animal models.

AIDS and Related Research 4 (ARRD)

Design and synthesis of compounds with potential for AIDS therapy; molecular modeling, molecular mechanics, and other structural and theoretical approaches in design of potential AIDS therapeutics; preclinical toxicologic, pharmacologic, pharmacokinetics, and metabolic aspects of drug development concerned with AIDS therapy; understanding biological and biochemical processes of HIV infection and maturation to find inhibitors of these processes (HIV-induced enzymes and structural proteins); mechanistic exploration with existing AIDS therapeutics to design improved entities; development of prodrug approaches and novel drug delivery vehicles; immunologic studies (drug discovery and development).

AIDS and Related Research 5 (ARRE)

Clinical therapy trials (in humans); pathology (pathological changes in human patients); opportunistic infections (molecular biologic and genetic studies on *Pneumocystis carinii*, *Toxoplasma gondii*, *Candida albicans*, *Cryptosporidium sp.*, *Crytococcus neoformans*, *Mycobacterium sp.*, and cytomegalovirus).

AIDS and Related Research 6 (ARRF)

Care provision/care providers; social support and family functioning; health, stress, and coping behavior; behavioral risk and behavioral modification; research design and implementation (strategies for securing behavioral or social data, methods of changing behavior, and procedures for assessment and analysis).

AIDS and Related Research 7 (ARRG)

Clinical neurology, neuropathology, neurophysiology, and neuropsychology (HIV-infected individuals or individuals at risk); sense systems (sensory function and sensory disorders related to HIV infection and AIDS).

Experimental Immunology (EI)

Tumor immunodiagnosis and immunotherapy; phagocytosis and antibody synthesis; immunopathogenesis; general immune response (biochemical aspects of tolerance, cell-mediated and humoral immunity, autoimmunity regulation, and developmental immunology).

Experimental Virology (EVR)

Viral diseases of man, lower animals, and plants; virus and cancer; cellular and molecular biology of viral replication (animal and plant); biochemistry of viral infections; biochemical–biophysical properties of viruses; classification and taxonomy of viruses.

Immunobiology (IMB)

Cellular and molecular immunology; immunogenetics (transplantation and tumor histocompatibility); tumor immunology (mechanisms of immune response to tumors); aging as an immune phenomenon.

Immunological Sciences (IMS)

Autoimmune disorders; humoral and cellular aspects of the immune response (tolerance *not* related to transplantation); hypersensitivity; immunologic status (assessment of immunologic parameters, mediators, immunopotentiators); developmental aspects of the immune response.

Immunology, Virology, and Pathology (IVP)

This panel reviews fellowship application in the areas of: immunology; virology; pathology of cardiovascular, renal, neurologic, respiratory diseases, and cancer.

Lung Physiology and Pathology (LBPA)

Lung cell culture and nonrespiratory lung function (isolation and characterization of lung cells in culture, biochemistry, and metabolism); airways (cellular, biochemical, and molecular biology of airways in health and disease including asthma and emphysema); pulmonary vasculature (effects of vasoactive agents, pulmonary hypertension, hypoxic pulmonary vasoconstriction, edema); surfactant and mucus (production, distribution, and clearance, role in lung pathology); immune function and disease of the lung (asthma, emphysema, bronchitis, fibrosis, cystic fibrosis, adult respiratory syndrome, pneumoconioses, e.g., anthracosis, silicosis, asbestosis, and other dust-induced diseases).

Pathology A (PTHA)

Anatomic areas (cardiovascular, renal, neurologic, and respiratory); pathophysiology (pathogenic changes in blood, urinary and tissue concentrations of enzymes and other chemical constituents); neuropathology (ultrastructural); immunopathology (tissue and serum changes associated with development of immune-sensitive systems); lung pathology (disease emphasis, e.g., anthracosis, silicosis, asbestosis, siderosis).

Pathology B (PATHB)

Oncological pathology (biology of cancer, tumor markers, receptors, oncogenes, regression, metastasis, metabolism of tumor cells, tumor diagnosis, cytogenetics); cellular pathology (morphologic changes in normal and tumor cells); immunopathology (emphasis on the tumor).

Virology (VR)

The same as EVR.

PHYSIOLOGICAL SCIENCES REVIEW SECTION

Biochemical Endocrinology (BCE)

Reproductive hormones; neuroendocrinology; mechanism of hormone action; end organ function; clinical (mechanism of action of sex hormones as therapeutic agents).

Epidemiology and Disease Control 1 (EDC-1)

Arthritic and rheumatoid diseases; osteoporosis; menopause; cardiovascular disease; diabetes; child growth; pregnancy and fertility; digestive and kidney diseases; measurement of incidence and prevalence of diseases; identification of risk factors;

development of research designs and methodologies; biostatistical methods; case–control studies; clinical trials and epidemiological studies.

Epidemiology and Disease Control 2 (EDC-2)

Cancer; infectious diseases; environmental and occupational risk factors; pulmonary diseases; sleep disorders; neurological disorders; measurement of incidence and prevalence of diseases; identification of risk factors; development of research designs and methodologies; biostatistical methods; case–control studies; clinical trials and epidemiological studies.

Endocrinology (END)

Neuroendocrinology; normal and abnormal function of the endocrine glands; hormone biosynthesis, metabolism, secretion, isolation, purification, and structure–function analysis; aging, growth, and other physiological processes (as applied to the endocrine system); mechanism of hormone action.

Experimental Therapeutics 1 (ET-1)

Drug development (antineoplastic); drug evaluation; biochemical pharmacology; cellular pharmacology; molecular pharmacology; molecular genetics (mechanism of action of antineoplastic agents and drug resistance); immunology (combined modalities of therapy); radiobiology (chemotherapy in combination with radiation); endocrinology (effects of chemotherapy on hormone-sensitive sites).

Experimental Therapeutics 2 (ET-2)

Drug evaluation; biochemical pharmacology (clinical); clinical investigations; biological response modifiers (cancer immunology studies in the clinic and in animals).

General Medicine B (GMB)

Endocrinology (related to water and electrolyte balance or mineral metabolism); water and electrolyte metabolism; skeletal system; urinary system; clinical disease, e.g., hypo- and hyperparathyroidism, hypo- and hypercalcemia, diabetes insipidus, metabolic acidosis and alkalosis, kidney stone pathophysiology, osteoporosis, rickets and normal and abnormal bone growth and development.

Human Embryology and Development 1 (HED-1)

Endocrinology of pregnancy; respiratory physiology; respiratory distress syndrome; sudden infant death syndrome; fetal-maternal cardiodynamics; pharmacology; parturition; pregnancy complications; diagnostic imaging; placental pathology; immunology of pregnancy; growth and development; fetal metabolism; computer modeling; molecular biology; placental transfer; toxicology (fetal and maternal).

Human Embryology and Development 2 (HED-2)

Embryology; cell biology; anatomy-morphology; genetics; teratology; biochemistry; embryo metabolism; molecular biology; developmental immunology; developmental neurology; placentation; electron microscopy; implantation; toxicology (embryonic).

Oral Biology and Medicine 1 (OBM-1)

Biochemistry/chemistry (connective tissue, saliva); dental materials; epidemiology and public health dentistry; oral microbiology/immunology; oral pathology; developmental biology and teratogenesis (pharmacological and hormonal changes and imbalances involved with craniofacial anomalies; clinical genetics related to orofacial dysfunctions and disfigurements); cell biology (oral soft tissue, salivary gland secretory mechanisms).

Oral Biology and Medicine 2 (OBM-2)

Anatomy/anthropology; biochemistry/chemistry (calcification, composition of teeth, bones, and periodontal tissues); biometry; mineralized tissue cell biology; dental materials (factors influencing chemical and physical properties of dental restorative materials); implantology (biological acceptance in the oral region); oral microbiology/immunology; oral pathology; oral surgery; behavior (treatment approaches to patients with pain).

Pharmacology (PHRA)

Cardiovascular (effects of drugs on the heart or cardiovascular system, cardiac glycosides, coronary vasodilators antiarrhythmics, antihypertensives); Drug metabolism (metabolic transformation of clinically active drugs in the mammalian system); pharmacokinetics; biopharmaceutics (drug bioavailability, drug dosage forms); clinical pharmacology (especially in the cardiovascular system).

Physiology (PHY)

Nervous system; muscle (morphology, electrical and mechanical activity); epithelial and cell membranes (mechanisms and kinetics of solute transport across biological membranes); model membranes (structure and physical chemistry, including of lipid bilayers).

Physiological Sciences (PSF)

This panel reviews fellowship applications in the areas of: endocrinology; reproductive and developmental sciences; muscle, renal, and bone physiology; pharmacology; toxicology; safety and occupational health; epidemiology; experimental therapeutics.

Reproductive Biology (REB)

Gonads (gametogenesis, gonad responses and functions, sperm capacitation); genital tract (histology and ultrastructure, zygote and gamete transport, hormone balance, immunologic phenomena, capacitation, placentation); fertility; endocrinology (chemistry and function of gonadal hormones); accessory organs of reproduction.

Reproductive Endocrinology (REN)

Endocrine functions of the mammary gland, ovary, testes, prostate, and uterus; problems in abnormal pediatric endocrinology; studies in contraception; problems of pregnancy related to hormone imbalance; management of endocrine disorders dealing with reproduction; studies of effects of environmental toxins on reproduction.

Safety and Occupational Health (SOH)

Epidemiologic studies (factors involved in the etiology of occupationally related diseases and injuries); toxicologic studies (toxic features in the work environment); industrial hygiene and engineering; occupational medicine and nursing (occupational health programs, medical records, employee assistance, health promotion); behavioral and motivational factors.

Toxicology 1 (TOX-1)

Biochemical toxicology; chemical carcinogenesis; clinical toxicology; genotoxicology (effects of toxicants on the germ cell; pathological states resulting from physical or chemical agents which are related to DNA repair/replication deficiencies); immunotoxicology (interaction of intoxicants with and effects on the immune system); hepatic/nephrotoxicology; xenobiotic metabolism.

Toxicology 2 (TOX-2)

Developmental and reproductive toxicology; heavy metal toxicology; inhalation/pulmonary toxicology; neurotoxicology; pesticide toxicology.

SPECIAL REVIEW SECTION

Special Emphasis Panel (SEP)

Applications for biomedical research technology resource grants, program projects (occasionally those assigned to NIGMS and NIDR), shared instrumentation grants, history of medicine, small business innovation grants, and applications that cannot be assigned to a "regular" study section as well as those that are math related.

Appendix 5

Institute Review Committee Referral Guidelines

MECHANISMS REVIEWED

- Program Projects (P01)
- Center Core Grants (P30)
- Specialized Center Grants (P50)
- Comprehensive Center Grants (P60)
- Cooperative Agreements (U01 and other U series)
- Institutional National Research Service Awards (T32)
- Academic Awards (K07)
- Clinical Investigator Awards (K08)
- Physician Scientist Awards (K11, K12)
- Fellowships (F32, F33)
- Conference Grants (R13)
- Research Demonstration Projects (R18)
- Contracts (N01)
- Minority Research Enhancement Program (MARC, MBRS, G12 etc.)

NATIONAL INSTITUTE ON AGING

Biological and Clinical Aging Review Committee (BCA)

This chartered review committee is subdivided into two subcommittees. Members are knowledgeable in the fields of molecular and cellular biology, immunology, biochemistry, animal science, pharmacology, internal medicine, behavioral medicine, nutrition, clinical assessment, and clinical epidemiology relevant to the process of aging.

Neuroscience, Behavior and Sociology of Aging Review Committee (NBSA)

This chartered review committee is subdivided into two subcommittees. Members are knowledgeable in the fields of Alzheimer's Disease, basic and clinical neuroscience, demography and survey design, psychology and behavior, and social sciences relevant to the process of aging.

NATIONAL INSTITUTE OF ALLERGY AND INFECTIOUS DISEASES

Allergy, Immunology and Transplantation Committee (AITC-1, AITC-2)

This committee is subdivided into two subcommittees.

Subcommittee 1 (AITC-1)

Clinical aspects of allergy and immunology, including immunopathology, infectious processes in immunologically mediated diseases, cellular immunology, immediate and delayed hypersensitivity, immune-mediated disorders, complement, antibodies, mechanisms of immunological disease, and immunodermatology.

Subcommittee 2 (AITC-2)

Basic aspects of immunology including transplantation biology, histocompatibility testing, transplantation immunology, immunochemistry, immunogenetics, cellular and molecular immunology, and lymphocyte biology.

Microbiology and Infectious Diseases Research Committee (MID)

Infectious diseases and the host response, including biology of infectious agents, pathogenesis and natural history, epidemiology and biometry, diagnosis, treatment and prevention, clinical trials, molecular microbiology, including recombinant nucleic acid molecular research, and mechanisms of resistance to antimicrobial agents.

Acquired Immunodeficiency Syndrome Research Review Committee (AIDS-1 to 4)

This committee deals with AIDS and its associated opportunistic infections and HTLV-III/LAV and related retroviruses and is divided into four subcommittees.

Basic Sciences Subcommittee (AIDS-1)

Immunology, including basic science studies in virology, immunology, and pathogenesis.

Clinical Applications, Prevention, and Treatment Subcommittee (AIDS-2)

Clinical applications; prevention; treatment.

Epidemiology and Technology Transfer Subcommittee (AIDS-3)

Epidemiology; technology transfer.

Basic Sciences II Subcommittee (AIDS-4)

Virology, including basic science studies in virology, immunology, pathogenesis.

NATIONAL INSTITUTE OF ARTHRITIS, MUSCULOSKELETAL AND SKIN DISEASES

Special Projects Review Committee (AMS)

Arthritis; muscle biology; musculoskeletal diseases; skin diseases.

NATIONAL CANCER INSTITUTE

Cancer Center Support Grant Review Committee (CCS)

Reviews applications for cancer center support grants in all areas relevant to cancer.

Cancer Clinical Investigation Review Committee (CCI)

Chemotherapy; radiation; surgery; immunotherapy; combined modality therapy.

Cancer Control Grant Review Committee (CCG)

Prevention; screening (detection); diagnosis; pretreatment (valuation); treatment; rehabilitation; continuing care activities.

Cancer Education Review Committee (CEC)

Cancer education; chronic disease prevention and cancer control; nutrition curricula development; short research experiences; training courses in response to specific announcements.

Cancer Research Manpower Review Committee (CT)

All areas relevant to cancer.

NATIONAL INSTITUTE OF DENTAL RESEARCH

Special Grants Review Committee (DSR)

All areas relevant to dental research.

NATIONAL INSTITUTE ON DEAFNESS AND OTHER COMMUNICATION DISORDERS

Communication Disorders Review Committee (CDRC)

All areas related to the mission of the NIDCD.

NATIONAL INSTITUTE OF DIABETES AND DIGESTIVE AND KIDNEY DISEASES

Diabetes and Digestive and Kidney Diseases Special Grants Review Committee (DDK)

This committee is subdivided into three subcommittees.

Subcommittee B (DDK-B)

Diabetes; endocrinology; metabolism.

Subcommittee C (DDK-C)

Digestive diseases; liver diseases; nutrition.

Subcommittee D (DDK-D)

Nephrology; urology; hematology.

NATIONAL INSTITUTE OF ENVIRONMENTAL HEALTH SCIENCES

Environmental Health Sciences Review Committee (EHS)

All areas relevant to the mission of the NIEHS.

NATIONAL EYE INSTITUTE

Vision Research Review Committee (VSN)

Retinal and choroidal diseases; corneal diseases; cataract; glaucoma; strabismus, amblyopia, and visual processing; collaborative clinical research.

NATIONAL INSTITUTE OF GENERAL MEDICAL SCIENCES

Cellular and Molecular Basis of Disease Review Committee (CMBD)

Multidisciplinary Predoctoral Training Grant applications (including MSTP) with primary emphasis in cellular, molecular, and developmental biology and biochemistry, including programs in genetics and structural biology. Postdoctoral Basic Pathobiology Training Grant applications.

Genetic Basis of Disease Review Committee (GBD)

Multidisciplinary Predoctoral Training Grant applications (including MSTP) with primary emphasis in genetics, including programs in cellular, molecular and developmental biology, and biotechnology. Postdoctoral Training Grant applications in genetics with emphasis on medical genetics.

Pharmacological Sciences Review Committee (PTR)

Interdisciplinary Predoctoral Training Grants (including MSTP) with primary emphasis on pharmacological sciences, including medicinal chemistry. Postdoctoral Research Training Grants in the areas of clinical pharmacology and anesthesiology.

Minority Programs Review Committee (MPRC)

This chartered review committee is subdivided into two subcommittees.

Minority Access to Research Career (MARC) Subcommittee A (MPRC-A)

All types of applications for MARC awards.

Minority Biomedical Research Support (MBRS) Subcommittee B (MPRC-B)

All types of applications for MBRS awards.

NATIONAL INSTITUTE OF CHILD HEALTH
AND HUMAN DEVELOPMENT

Maternal and Child Health Research Committee (HDMC)

Pregnancy and perinatology including physiology of pregnancy and fetal development, labor and birth, physiology of the newborn, sudden infant death syndrome, pediatric AIDS; genetics and teratology, including basic and clinical studies of normal development; developmental defects, including developmental and clinical genetics; developmental biology, including postimplantation embryonic development; teratology; developmental immunology; nutrition and endocrinology, including developmental nutrition, infant nutrition, gastrointestinal development, obesity, and nutritional antecedents of diabetes and other adult diseases, cultural and behavioral aspects of nutrition, physical growth, anthropometrics and nutritional status, developmental endocrinology, developmental neuroendocrinology, pediatric endocrinology, diabetes mellitus, including preventive, psychosocial, genetic and immunological aspects; behavioral development, including developmental behavioral biology (developmental psychobiology), communicative processes (speech, language and reading, dyslexia), learning, cognition, perception, and memory; social and affective development, illness-related and health-related behaviors; behavioral pediatrics; developmental behavioral neurobiology.

Mental Retardation Research Committee (HDMR)

Developmental neurobiological studies; inborn errors of metabolism and endocrinology; genetic/cytogenetic disorders associated with MR; molecular biology; gene therapy; toxicology, nutrition, and environmental factors in etiology, treatment and prevention; developmental pharmacology and psychopharmacology; infectious diseases in etiology, prevention and treatment; diagnosis; perinatal factors; psychobiological and psychological processes; early interventions for infants born at risk; educational intervention; behavioral analysis of MR individuals; family and community studies; language and communication in MR individuals; cognition and learning in MR individuals; behavior in residential and educational settings; socioecological processes; epidemiology of MR.

Population Research Committee (HDPR)

Reproductive sciences, including reproductive physiology of male and female; reproductive biology; reproductive endocrinology; reproductive neuroendocrinology; reproductive biochemistry; reproductive molecular biology; obstetrics/gynecology of reproduction; reproductive medicine; cell structure and ultrastructure related to reproduction; male and female reproduction; preimplantation embryonic development. Population sciences, including sociology, demography, economic studies related to population research; psychology related to population research; sexuality and fertility-related behavior.

NATIONAL HEART, LUNG, AND BLOOD INSTITUTE

Clinical Trials Review Committee (CLTR)

Multicenter cooperative trials related to the NHLBI mission.

Heart, Lung, and Blood Research Review Committee (HLBA)

Cardiovascular diseases; cardiovascular physiology; lung diseases; pulmonary physiology; cardiopulmonary transplantation; biomedical engineering and devices; behavioral medicine.

Heart, Lung, and Blood Research Review Committee (HLBB)

Atherosclerosis and arteriosclerosis; hypertension including related kidney involvement; blood research including hematology, physiology of normal and abnormal blood, blood banking, blood diseases.

Research Manpower Committee (MR)

All areas related to the NHLBI mission.

NATIONAL LIBRARY OF MEDICINE

Biomedical Library Review Committee (BLR)

Medical informatics (computers in medicine); medical (health sciences) libraries; medical knowledge utilization; medical knowledge organization; integrated academic information management systems.

NATIONAL INSTITUTE OF NEUROLOGICAL DISORDERS AND STROKE

Neurological Disorders Program Project Review A Committee (NSPA)

Demyelinating diseases, including multiple sclerosis; motoneuron disease, including amyotrophic lateral sclerosis; parkinsonism and other involuntary movement disorders; pain; stroke; trauma to the nervous system (head and spinal cord); neural regeneration; sleep disorders.

Neurological Disorders Program Project Review B Committee (NSPB)

Basic neurosciences; degenerating/dementing/demyelinating disorders such as myasthenia gravis, AIDS dementia and multiple sclerosis; degenerative disorders of muscle including muscular dystrophy; epilepsy and other convulsive disorders; neural development including Huntington's disease; neural plasticity; neurotransmitter studies.

Training Grant and Career Development Review Committee (NST)

All areas related to the mission of the NINDS.

NATIONAL CENTER FOR RESEARCH RESOURCES

Animal Resources Review Committee (AR)

Laboratory animal medicine; animal resources; animal models; primatology.

Biotechnology Resources Review Committee (BRC)

Areas related to the Biomedical Research Technology program.

General Clinical Research Centers Committee (CLR)

Center applications and supplements and research projects related to centers (R24).

NATIONAL CENTER FOR HUMAN GENOME RESEARCH

Genome Research Review Committee (GRRC)

Construction of high-resolution genetic linkage maps; development of a variety of physical maps; determination of the complete nucleotide sequence of the DNA of selected organisms; development of the capability of collecting, storing, distributing, and analyzing the data and materials produced; development of appropriate new technologies and interpretation of the information produced; and issues related to the ethical, legal, and social implications of the Human Genome Initiative.

NATIONAL CENTER FOR NURSING RESEARCH

Nursing Science Research Review Committee (NRRC)

Basic and clinically oriented research to improve patient care; promotion of health and prevention of illness; understanding of individual family and community responses to acute and chronic illnesses and disabilities; and the ethics of patient care.

References

Allen, E.M. 1960. Why are research grants disapproved? *Science* 132:1532–1534.

Cuca, J.M. 1983. NIH grant applications for clinical research: Reasons for poor ratings or disapproval. *Clin. Res.* 31:453–461.

Department of Health and Human Services. 1983. *Protection of human subjects.* Code of Federal Regulations, 45 CFR 46.

Division of Research Grants, National Institutes of Health. 1991. *Activity Codes, Organizational Codes, and Definitions Used in Extramural Programs.*

———— 1991. *DRG Peer Review Trends.*

———— 1990. *DRG Peer Review Trends: Member Characteristics.*

———— 1991. *Extramural Trends FY 1981–1990.*

———— 1987. *Handbook for Executive Secretaries.*

———— 1990. *Helpful Hints on Preparing a Fellowship Application to the National Institutes of Health.*

———— 1990. *Helpful Hints on Preparing a Research Grant Application to the National Institutes of Health.*

Gordon, S. L. and Watson, D. M. 1990. Use and importance of the NIH noncompeting continuation application. *FASEB J.* 4:2438–2440.

Office for Protection from Research Risks. 1986. *Public Health Service Policy on Humane Care and Use of Laboratory Animals.*

Office of Management and Budget. 1991. Circular A-21.

———— 1987. Circular A-122.

Office of Science Policy and Legislation. 1991. *NIH Data Book.*

Wright, S. 1971. Reasons for Disapproval of National Institutes of Health Research Project Grant Applications. Unpublished.

Index